SURVIVING CANCER
EMOTIONALLY

SURVIVING CANCER EMOTIONALLY

Learning How to Heal

ROGER GRANET, M.D.

John Wiley & Sons, Inc.

New York • Chichester • Weinheim • Brisbane • Singapore • Toronto

Design and production by Navta Associates, Inc.

This publication is designed to provide accurate and authoritative information in regard to the subject matter covered. It is sold with the understanding that the publisher is not engaged in rendering professional services. If professional advice or other expert assistance is required, the services of a competent professional person should be sought.

The anecdotal information included in the book is based on composites or hypothetical individuals. Any similarities between the case study description and actual persons are purely coincidental.

Library of Congress Cataloging-in-Publication Data:

Granet, Roger.
    Surviving cancer emotionally : learning how to heal / Roger Granet.
        p. cm.
    Includes index.
    ISBN: 0-471-38741-X (paper : alk. paper)
    1. Cancer—Psychological aspects.   I. Title.

RC262 .G7325   2001
362. 1'96994'0019—dc21   2001026450

Printed in the United States of America

10 9 8 7 6 5 4 3 2 1

To Valerie, Courtney, and Jamie
With boundless love

And

To Lois and Lester Granet
and Ruth and Joseph Waters
With endless warmth

CONTENTS

ACKNOWLEDGMENTS

I wish to thank my agent, Judith Riven, whose belief in this project and wisdom along the way provided the energy and guidance for its fruition; Elizabeth Zack, my editor at John Wiley & Sons, for her encouragement and creativity, as well as her assistant, Kellam Ayres; Robert Aquinas McNally for the enormity of his exquisite talent and acumen; Kim Nir for her remarkable abilities; Laurie Martin for her efforts and patience; Dr. Clifford Taylor for his constant support, Drs. Jimmie Holland, Bill Breitbart, and Mary Jane Massie of Memorial Sloan-Kettering Cancer Center for their seminal scholarship and warm collegiality; numerous oncologists, especially Drs. Ken Adler, Bill DeRosa, Chuck Farber, Gary Gerstein, and Steve Papish, who blend humanity with superb clinical and medical knowledge; Robin Matthews for her kind assistance; the oncology and psychiatry nursing staffs at Morristown Memorial, New York Presbyterian, and Memorial Sloan-Kettering hospitals for their skillful hearts; and my mentors, Drs. Arnold Cooper and John Talbott, for being such generous role models.

I also want to express my appreciation to Jamie, Courtney, Valerie, Lois Granet, Jack Cohen, Michael Raff, Ruth Waters, Gail Granet Velez, Vicki and William Semel, Hank and Gerry Alpert, Peter and Camille Ehrenberg, Carol and Larry Gelber, and Jill and Jerry Wichtel. Their goodness sustains me.

Finally, I am honored to acknowledge the many patients and their families who have permitted me to participate in their courageous journeys.

INTRODUCTION

CANCER. This diagnosis brings a deluge of complex emotions. Uncertainty, fear of suffering and death, anxiety over the prospect of therapies that may prove as hard to bear as the disease itself, an overwhelming sense of powerlessness and loss of control of life not yet lived fully. Cancer may arise in the breast or colon or lung, or elsewhere, but its effects reach beyond the involved tissues to trouble the mind as well.

Over the past several decades, medical research on the physical aspects of cancer has advanced our understanding of the disease and increased our ability to treat it. Some forms of cancer have become much more curable, and treatment has reached a new level of sophistication and selectivity. Still, there is more to treating cancer than the technologies of chemotherapy, surgery, and radiation. The psychological side of cancer, which plays a key role in dealing successfully with the disease, is the subject of this book.

Surviving Cancer Emotionally springs from two sources of information. One is the growing medical literature on cancer's emotional face, a burgeoning field known as psycho-oncology. The other is my own experience as a psycho-oncologist, a physician trained as a psychiatrist who specializes in the treatment of cancer patients. For more than twenty years, I have been privileged to spend a part of each day with people who have cancer.

In all these years of dealing with the disease, I have developed tremendous awe and respect for cancer—clearly not because of the suffering it

1

causes or its biologically potent cellular madness but for its potential to change lives. Cancer delivers a loud wake-up call. It provides an opportunity to review and rewrite existence, and it demands that we look at this lease called life. When an individual faces cancer, the powerful emotional consequences of the disease permits him or her to examine life very closely; to pay attention to inner experience, relationships, the past, the future, and—most important—the present. Once diagnosed with cancer, a person is never the same. The disease creates a mandate for change.

What dazzles me about cancer is how many patients use their illness as a chance to stretch and grow. Over the years, the potent stories of my cancer patients' lives have become even more compelling. And as we converse during office psychotherapy sessions, consultations on oncology units, or late-night phone calls, I realize that my patients have taught me as much as I have taught them.

Those many lessons began early in my career, and they have shaped my development as a physician and as a person. I had been aware from the first days of my medical training that I wanted to be a psychiatrist. The symptoms of disease interested me far less than the emotional issues facing the people who were suffering from them. Surgery, for example, held so little intrigue for me that I once fell asleep while assisting in a gallbladder removal. I wanted to know more about the patient's *unconscious* and not the unconscious patient. This desire took a specific focus around cancer during the last year of my psychiatric residency at The Payne Whitney Psychiatric Clinic at the NY Hospital–Cornell Medical Center.

Late one night, an intern asked me to see an elderly man who had just had a cancer successfully removed from his brain. The patient was agitated, most likely from the high doses of steroids needed to reduce postoperative swelling. I calmed him down with a lot of reassurance and a little medication.

The next morning when I returned to see how he was feeling, he appeared much more at ease. We began to talk. He told me about his life's work as a law school professor and about the love he felt for his garden, the pleasure he took in tending to nature. Then, as I got up to leave his room, he looked up at me, still in a somewhat confused state, and said, "I don't know what you do, but you seem to have a very curious job."

Without thinking, I answered, "I'm a psychiatrist who loves to work with people who have cancer."

I had said it for the first time. In the years since then, I have said it to myself many more times, as I have watched people with the disease grow, stretch, and deepen emotionally. In a way, this book is written as a thank-you note to the many patients who have taught me. Their tenacious work to find meaning in living, during the crisis of illness, has given me boundless gifts of insight into the human spirit. Cancer teaches that today's experiences, relationships, longings, and loves cannot be put off until tomorrow. Existence is brief—a reality of which people with cancer are much more aware than the rest of us. Most learn to embrace the pain and joy of their moments with renewed vigor despite the fear, uncertainty, and lack of control that are also the inescapable realities of serious disease.

There is another basic reason for understanding cancer's emotional aspect. Effective coping—that is, coming to terms with the disease emotionally and marshalling one's resources in the face of it—greatly affects quality of life, with or without serious illness. In its own way, good mental health is an antidote against the rigorous trials of cancer diagnosis, treatment, and survivorship. Understanding the predictable emotional cycles of cancer and learning how to deal with them is a key aspect of treating the disease. This is healing—achieving wholeness and integrity in the face of cancer.

Much of this book offers information: It tells you what to expect. It unravels the tangled, difficult feelings that surround cancer—emotions that can make patients and those close to them feel overwhelmed—and shows them often to be the normal reactions of an individual facing a crisis. Then it details effective ways of dealing with these feelings. Knowing what one is up against and realizing that help is available are key elements of effective coping. And should emotional reactions themselves become troubling and abnormal, appropriate psychiatric intervention can help greatly.

This book opens by describing common emotional reactions to the diagnosis of cancer and looks a the importance of strengthening—and, at times, developing—the coping skills critical to living life in the face of cancer. After disproving the popular misconception that individuals cause their own cancers by responding poorly to stress, the book then explores the connection between coping skills, quality of life, and even disease outcome. Suggestions and specific advice on coping are detailed. The spectrum of emotions that the disease can trigger, ranging from mild anxiety and sadness to severe panic and depression, are explored. Next, the book focuses on the predictable cycles of feelings surrounding specific stages: diagnosis; treatments such as chemotherapy, radiation, and surgery; remission; and survivorship. Psychiatric and neurological disorders that can appear as effects of certain cancers or side effects of treatment are also discussed. The impact cancer has on family and friends is covered in a separate chapter. Of course, no book about cancer would be complete without dealing with death and dying, which are discussed repeatedly in these pages and more closely in Chapter 6. In closing, the book details the significant lessons cancer can teach about a life laced with greater meaning—sorrows put into perspective, joys more fully felt.

Cancer provides a powerful journey that kindles every aspect of our being and offers us a chance for feeling the depth of our experiences in each and every moment. It shouts at us to look straight in the eye at life. I hope this book does the same.

PART ONE

CANCER AND FEELINGS

1

UNDERSTANDING THE EMOTIONAL AND PHYSICAL REALITIES OF CANCER

THE HOUSE I GREW UP IN was a good place to get sick—up to a point. When I came down with a cold or flu, nurturance enveloped me like a warm blanket. To be ill was to be cared for. My mother prepared my favorite meal every time I asked for it: peanut butter and jelly on rye toast with the crust cut off. My father, dressed in a business suit from his day as an accountant, came to my bed bearing every brand and flavor of cough drop in one hand and a stack of *Archie* and *Superman* comics in the other.

Life-threatening illness, though, occasioned another response. When I was twelve, my mother's sister, Hazel, developed cancer. I had no sense of what the word *cancer* meant or any idea of what to do about the appearance of this disease in my family. Anxiety over this caused me to ask endless questions, yet my parents sidestepped my queries or ignored them altogether. Clearly, they wanted to avoid any discussion of what cancer was and what it meant for Hazel and her family. And when we visited my aunt through the years of her illness, that avoidance blossomed inside me as fright and helplessness.

In my family, commonplace sickness invited openness, support, love, and ease. But when disease crossed a certain line, it became feared. Unconsciously I came to know that life-threatening illnesses evoke a different set of psychological responses in family and friends.

My family was hardly different from most other families. Colds, flu, a hospital stay for surgery, and broken bones prompt outpourings of sympathy, offers of assistance, flowers, and get-well cards. With an illness that can kill, the cards and flowers may also come, but things are different. Denial, rationalization—that is, trying to justify the diagnosis—and often rigidity take the place of openness, truth, and flexibility.

This phenomenon hits home with cancer. No disease is more deeply and profoundly feared. Cancer symbolizes the inevitability of dying, death, and pain. A cancer diagnosis brings the individual and his or her family face-to-face with the reality that we all may suffer and we all will die.

Denial—the conscious or unconscious statement that "this isn't really what I fear it is"—builds a collusion of silence around cancer. People don't even want to say the word, as if pronouncing it makes the disease more real than it already is. They want to put a distance between themselves and anything so obviously fearful. Patients aren't the only ones; physicians do this too. Again and again, I have heard doctors refer to cancer as the "big C." In the New York City area, there's an ongoing medical joke of referring to Memorial Sloan-Kettering Cancer Center as the "Home of the Mets"—a pun linking nearby Shea Stadium, where the Mets play baseball, with *metastasis,* the technical term that refers to spreading cancer.

The level of popular and professional denial shows how deeply cancer involves the emotions. Yet the denial does us no good. The only way to begin to understand cancer as a disease is to call it what it is, to tear down the wall of silence, close the distance between ourselves and the disease, say the word out loud, and admit the feelings it raises.

When Cells Go Awry

The first step toward tearing down the wall is to understand cancer for what it is. Cancer is a disease—that is, a deviation or interruption in the ordinary structure or function of an organ. Cancer begins at the body's most basic level: the cell. That much we know. But we are unsure of just what causes cancer to occur. Apparently, there is some kind of dynamic interaction between an individual's genetic complement—what he or she inherited—and environmental factors, such as diet and exposure to toxins. In other words, there is no one single cause of cancer. Rather, a variety of different internal and external characteristics come together and affect the basic cellular level of the body.

According to one leading idea, the change that leads to cancer occurs in the mechanism of cell growth and development. When cells are developing in the embryo before birth, many are undifferentiated—that is, they have the potential to become almost any part of the body. Then, as they develop and differentiate, cells become one thing or another—for example, bone, or part of the brain, or the lining of the lung. Differentiation defines the growth and functions of the cell, as well as its life span. After a definite length of time, the cell dies and is usually replaced. Essentially, we are constantly being recycled. At the cellular level, none of us is the man or woman he or she was five years ago.

In cancer something goes wrong with cell growth. Unlike normal cells, whose growth and life span are limited, cancer cells don't stop dividing when they reach a specified size, and they look more like undifferentiated cells than the differentiated cells in the surrounding tissue. As a result, they continue to expand, push into surrounding cells, and destroy or replace them. Many cancers release secretions that prompt blood vessels to grow into them, providing them with a richer supply of nutrients than what neighboring normal cells receive. And cancer cells don't stay put. As they invade the vessels that carry blood and lymph, they are carried into distant parts of the body. They may lodge in other tissues, and, if they survive attack by white blood cells, they can attach to the new site and start growing and dividing. This is metastasis—cancer's propensity to move from one site to another.

Some cancer researchers believe the disease is a malfunction of the immune system. According to this hypothesis, cancer cells are being produced all the time, but they are quickly detected and destroyed by the immune system, particularly by natural killer (NK) cells. Cancer takes hold when something interferes with the immune system and undercuts the effectiveness of the NK attack. Some of the abnormal cells survive, take hold, grow, and begin to spread.

Technically, a cancer is a malignant neoplasm. *Neoplasm* refers to any new, abnormal growth. *Malignant* refers to cancer's propensity to lack differentiation, grow, multiply, invade, and spread. In contrast, a benign, or noncancerous, tumor is less likely to penetrate neighboring cells and tissues, to migrate from one body part to another, or to interfere with the body's healthy structure and function.

One of my physician friends refers to cancer cells as adolescents. Why? They haven't grown up yet, they don't know when to stop, they act out, and they're unruly and ill-behaved! The difference is that if you wait long enough, adolescents grow up all by themselves and become mature individuals. In the case of cancer, waiting around means that the cancer continues to grow and remains part of your body.

The symptoms of cancer come first from the neoplasm's growth, which can press on nerves and cause malfunction and pain, block passageways such as the intestine, cause bleeding in internal organs, and push aside normally functioning cells. For example, as a liver cancer grows and takes over from healthy tissue, more and more normal liver function is lost, and various kinds of metabolic problems arise. In addition, with their rich supply of blood vessels and potent capacity to divide, cancers act like internal parasites, using up energy that normally would have been directed elsewhere. The result can be diminished appetite, weight loss, extreme fatigue, and, in advanced cases, a wasted look to the body.

The rationale behind the various kinds of cancer treatments draws from scientific knowledge of how cancer progresses. Surgery is useful, particularly before the cancer has metastasized to distant sites, because it removes the malignant neoplasm. Radiation and chemotherapy "poison" cells as they divide. Since cancer cells grow so much faster than normal cells, they are particularly vulnerable to this kind of attack. Since some cancers are hormone-dependent (they grow faster in the presence of certain hormones), removing, blocking, or adding hormones may greatly slow the cancer's growth and eliminate or reduce its symptoms. And a newer treatment called immunotherapy focuses on mobilizing the body's own immune system to fight the cancer.

Where Feelings Come into Play

In the past thirty years, cancer treatment has become vastly more sophisticated, selective, and effective. Interestingly, as physicians have become more and more skilled at managing the disease, they have also come to understand the important role emotions play in the entire cancer process. Once we thought that the body, where cancer cells run riot, and the mind or psyche, where emotions happen, were separate spheres. Now we know that they are but two manifestations of the same single being. Medicine can't treat one without addressing the other.

There was a time when most physicians didn't even tell patients what they had. They used euphemistic words such as "growth" or "mass" and consigned the patient to "God's hands." Then, about forty years ago, physicians came to understand that withholding information from the patient or telling a lie undercut the trust the patient felt for the physician and was inherently destructive. More and more physicians began telling patients the truth about their condition. This revelation worked to the benefit of both patient and physician. Patients were better able to talk meaningfully with their doctors and take part in decisions about their treatment, while physicians no longer had to wrestle with truth issues.

At about the same time, Dr. Elisabeth Kübler-Ross's work on open communication with dying patients, many of them succumbing to cancer, led to a new insight into the importance of the psyche in facing serious illness and death. Increasingly, too, psychiatrists began working as consultants with other physicians treating cancer patients, particularly those affected by anxiety, depression, and delirium. This movement led to the development of the psychiatric specialty known as psycho-oncology, which studies how emotions and personality affect the experience of disease, how cancer alters the psychology of patients and their loved ones, and how patients can shift thought and behavior, often with the help of a professional, to enhance the quality of their lives.

In erasing the artificial barrier between mind and body and in learning how to treat cancer patients as whole beings, we have come to a number of key understandings. For one, there is no such thing as a cancer personality. Popular thinking—fostered in fact by some now-discredited research—has held that certain personality traits contribute to cancer. In a way, this idea isn't particularly revolutionary. It has long been known that driven, high-performing people—so-called type A personalities—are more prone to heart disease than are more relaxed individuals. It is also known that depression slows or impairs the immune system. Wouldn't it make sense, therefore, that certain personality traits can result in cancer?

One theory, unsupported by scientific data, is the so-called type C, or cancer-prone, personality—the individual who, almost directly opposite to type A, is appeasing, unassertive, socially compliant, and unwilling or unable to express resentment, anger, and other negative emotions. As yet, there is no solid research to show any clear connection between personality and the onset of cancer. People of different personality types get cancer with equal frequency. In addition, experiences known to produce symptoms similar to depression do not result in cancer any more often than would be expected otherwise. Reliable studies show that while people who have lost a spouse are at a heightened risk of death within a year of that loss, the increase in fatalities comes from causes other than cancer, such as heart disease and accidents. Cancer is no more widespread among bereaved people than among any group of similar age, ethnic background, and socioeconomic status. Based on what we now know, personality factors and stressful life events do not significantly affect the onset of cancer.

Indeed, the notion that personality can cause cancer has a destructive effect on people who get the disease: It essentially blames the patient for being ill. The argument suggests the patient can have complete control over cancer by purging his or her mind and heart of negative thoughts and feelings and replacing them with positive ones. There is no evidence that this is true. Like the unproven notion of type C as the cancer personality, this mind-over-matter belief subjects people to guilt feelings for being unable to cure their cancer despite concerted efforts to engage in nothing but positive thinking.

Even though there is no proof that a person's emotional structure causes cancer, it may affect disease progression. There is strong evidence that emotional well-being improves quality of life during cancer and may even extend survival time. While the scientific studies in this area are not conclusive, they are suggestive.

A research team led by Steven Greer, M.D., of the University of London, looked at the connection between personality styles and survival with breast cancer. Results of the research suggested that women exhibiting what the research team called a fighting spirit lived longer than did those who were stoically accepting of their condition or whose moods mixed hopelessness with helplessness. The number of patients Greer and his colleagues studied is too small to draw firm conclusions, and the research failed to control for the stage of the cancer, which is a crucial variable in predicting survival time. Still, this research suggests that a determined approach can help in fighting the disease. (*Note:* It's important to keep in mind, however, that different people fight in different ways. Some are quietly determined, whereas others are loud, angry, and fierce. Since we all have different personalities, there is no one-size-fits-all fighting spirit. Don't feel guilty about *how* you fight your illness; rather, commit yourself to fighting in the way *you* find most fitting.)

Another intriguing research effort at Stanford University headed by David Spiegel, M.D., focused on the effects of therapy for patients with advanced breast cancer. Some of the patients in the study received standard medical treatment alone, while others were given group therapy along with training in self-hypnosis for pain. After one year, the patients receiving therapy and hypnosis training reported fewer disturbances in mood, more energy, and less pain that did those undergoing standard medical treatment alone. Even more curiously, the therapy group on average lived more than twice as long as the medical care group. Dr. Spiegel suggests that the ability to express feelings in the group therapy session, the sense of acceptance by other patients and the medical staff, and the ability to seek out answers to problems may have led to better self-care. Currently, additional research is being undertaken with breast cancer patients at Stanford and elsewhere to see if the same connection between therapy, improved quality of life, and longer survival can be demonstrated.

Research in the emerging field of psychoimmunology underscores the direct connection between mind and body and shows further how emotional response to cancer may affect the disease. The brain not only is the seat of emotions, but it also has powerful links to the immune system, so feelings can affect the way the immune system responds. Psychologist

Sandra Levy and her co-workers at the National Cancer Institute and the University of Pittsburgh found that cancer patients who felt socially sup-ported by others demonstrated increased activity by natural killer (NK) cells, which distinguish cancer cells from healthy cells and attack them. Research by Fawzy I. Fawzy, M.D., and his colleagues at the UCLA School of Medicine found that when malignant melanoma patients receiving psychotherapy reported a decrease in depression and anxiety, their immune system activity increased.

As we will see in Chapter 2, which focuses on the skills needed to cope with cancer, there is no simple and easy formula for mobilizing emotional resources to fight the disease. Still, given what we now know, it appears that patients who understand what happens emotionally during cancer and who are offered good psychological resources can greatly improve the quality of their lives, and, although they may not be able to stop their dis-ease, they may possibly slow its progression.

Emotional Reactions to Cancer

A diagnosis of cancer brings forth one's fundamental fears, which are based on equally fundamental illusions. The first concerns death. Practi-cally no one really believes that he or she is going to die one of these days. The event seems to exist so far off in a distant future that its inevitability appears merely theoretical, yet the diagnosis of cancer turns the theoreti-cal future into the threatening present. When told they have cancer, most patients immediately ask some version of the big question: "So, is this going to kill me?" (fearing of course that it will). The reality of death has just torn through the illusion of immortality. The emotional consequences are profound.

The second emotional reaction centers around losing control. As soon as one receives a cancer diagnosis, he or she is drawn into a strange world of doctors, hospitals, complex medical terminology, and tests and thera-pies that range from uncomfortable and unpleasant to life-altering. Sud-denly the individual goes from a man or woman who runs his or her own life to a patient whose life is dictated by larger forces over which he or she has little control. In fact, none of us really controls life, but no one understands the absurdity of this illusion more deeply and immediately than someone who has been diagnosed with cancer.

The third emotional response is uncertainty. Before cancer, most people had what they considered a reasonable idea about their appearance and overall health, and how the future was shaping up. Cancer cancels that certainty and replaces it with a long list of I-don't-knows.

The fear of death, the loss of control, and the introduction of uncertainty underlie the emotional reactions to cancer. Cancer poses a direct threat to life and autonomy as real and as physical as the cold-blooded thug stepping out of a dark alley with a pistol pointed at your heart. The reactions are largely what you might expect: fear, anxiety, depression, anger, panic. At best, the experience is disconcerting. At worst, it may seem more devastating than the disease.

The first step in dealing with the emotional reality of cancer is understanding the normal cycles of emotions that characterize the course of the disease. If you have just received a cancer diagnosis and you find your nights are filled with anxious thoughts of long, slow, lingering death, you are not alone. This reaction is absolutely typical. But by knowing what to expect, you can begin to mobilize the needed inner and outer resources. This book will help you understand the normal emotional complications of cancer and show you ways of dealing with them. It will also explore what to do when reactions are beyond the norm.

The next step is to prepare yourself for something unusual about cancer: the way it calls into question how you have lived your life up to the present. In a manner more profound that any other life-threatening disease, cancer forces a reevaluation of the past and the present. It may, in fact, lead you to change fundamental aspects of the way you have been in the world. You may set out to create a new future.

Nancy, a pediatric nurse and the mother of adolescent twin boys, was in her mid-forties when I first saw her as a patient. The impression she gave was of a warm, sweet woman who moved through life intent on not ruffling feathers or making noise. She was the youngest of three children and the only daughter of a strict, demanding father and a shy, passive mother.

Nancy emulated her mother's quiet, pleasing ways, and she worked hard to satisfy her father, who set a person's worth by external accomplishment alone. Nancy had been an excellent student, yet her father had largely overlooked her successes to lavish praise on her two older brothers, who were outgoing, gregarious athletes. No matter what she did, Nancy felt she lived in their shadow.

Nancy earned a degree in nursing, specialized in pediatrics, and was a success in her career, not so much as someone who climbed the medical hierarchy but as a healer to whom patients gravitated for her soft, motherly ways. She was well liked, in part because she was too agreeable to confront even people she disliked, in part because she was warm, kind, generous, and always smiling. Since Nancy hated the spotlight, she sometimes felt that the more ambitious of her peers piggybacked off her success, but she became good at denying that those feelings existed and at explaining them away when they became too obvious to ignore.

Nancy was much the same in her family life. Her husband was the strong, silent type, who provided well, enjoyed his status as patriarch, and, though loving, never encouraged Nancy to talk about herself. Instead, she took care of him in every way. She was a nurturing mother to her twins, always ready with home-baked cookies and a willing ear. Although by nature a worrier, Nancy kept her concerns to herself and paid little attention to her own needs and desires.

In short, Nancy asked for little from life and expected less. Her job, as she saw it, was to do for others. Never particularly self-reflective, she seemed to embrace her roles as nurse, mother, wife, and caretaker.

At first, the pain Nancy experienced in her lower abdomen did nothing to disrupt the structure of her life. However, the discomfort, dull and annoying, wouldn't go away. Soon it was accompanied by burning sensations when she urinated. During a routine Pap smear, she mentioned the problem to her gynecologist, who referred her to a urologist. The results of the long series of tests surprised Nancy: bladder cancer.

"But, you know, I didn't really feel that upset," she confessed to me later. "I had some trouble sleeping for a few nights, and sometimes my heart would race, but then I told myself, 'Look, it's early stage. This is no big deal. Grin and bear it.' So I did."

Surgery to remove a portion of her bladder was successful, and Nancy recovered relatively quickly, with no complications from the operation. So far, so good. Then her oncologist ordered a series of chemotherapy cycles, a treatment sometimes used in Nancy's type of cancer.

With its accompanying nausea, fatigue, and hair loss, chemotherapy brought the reality of cancer home to Nancy. The loss of control, the uncertainty about her future, and the fear of suffering and death broke through her well-constructed defenses of denial and rationalization. Maybe this was early-stage cancer, and maybe her prognosis was excellent, but she felt like something the cat dragged in nonetheless. Her mood shifted from always smiling to ever sad. Long crying spells beset her, particularly in the early mornings, when her spirits dropped especially low. Things that used to be the center of her life lost most of their interest. She had no desire to connect sexually with her husband, no energy to read romance novels—which had been her preferred form of entertainment— and too little patience to listen to the many ups and downs of her twins' adolescent lives. Her thinking was slow, unreliable and constantly negative, so she took a long leave of absence from work, even though nursing had always sustained her. Nancy felt eternally tired and was tempted to stay in bed most of the time, but sleep came only irregularly and in short, unsatisfying snatches.

"I'd sit awake downstairs at night and think about dying. Sometimes I saw myself dead. I was a corpse amid banks of flowers, and my family was coming to pay last respects. I thought it was a dream, then I'd pinch myself and I'd know I was awake. This was my life. It was horrible to dream about," she told me later.

One of the nurses in the oncologist's office where Nancy was receiving chemotherapy recognized how low she was and passed that information on to her doctor, who made an appointment for Nancy to see me.

"I didn't have enough energy to say no," she said.

Nancy's emotional predicament was hardly unique. Faced with serious disease, many cancer patients drop into depression. For some, the experience is mild, and they are able to shake off the low mood in time. For a substantial number, however, the mood change is more profound. This was the case with Nancy, who had a significant depression. Fortunately, depression can be treated effectively and successfully. In Nancy's case, I recommended psychotherapy for a few months, an antidepressant, and an antianxiety medication to help her relax at night and sleep.

Without doubt, cancer precipitated Nancy's depression. Yet I suspected that there was more to her suffering than this serious disease. The first glimmer of that reality came during our fourth visit together, when I asked her if the antidepressant, which can require several weeks to take effect, was helping.

Instead of answering in her usual short, polite monosyllables, Nancy said, "Oh, I do feel somewhat better—less dark, less shaky. But I still have this sense that I'm nothing more than a failure. The pills aren't doing anything about that."

I recognized that she was working toward some feelings hidden deep inside her. I wanted to hear more, hoping that as she gave these feelings words, she would recognize them as her own. "But why is that?" I said. "You're doing well with the cancer. Everything is going fine."

"My oncologist says that too. She says I'm doing just great. But for someone who's doing so great, I can't do what I'm supposed to be doing," Nancy explained. "I feel useless." Tears formed in the corners of her eyes.

"Useless? What do you mean by useless?" I asked.

"I can't do what I'm supposed to do." She was nearly shouting, her voice high and tight with frustration. "I don't have any hair. I don't have any energy. I'm just a middle-aged woman with cancer who can't be the wife and mother I should be. I have no value in my family."

"You're right about your physical condition. But it's *temporary.* You will get better when the chemotherapy is over. So, why does being sick mean you have no value?"

Nancy sat quietly and turned the question over in her mind. Tears tumbled down her cheeks. The core of sadness in her was breaking through. Finally she said, "I guess I only experience a feeling of worth when I can do for others."

"Do you feel that you're worth being done for too?" I asked.

Again she was very still. Minutes passed, and the tears continued to stream down her face. "I guess I never thought so. Not from the time I was a girl. The only time I felt like I had a right to take up my space on the earth was when I was doing something for my father, my mother, my brothers. Now it's my husband and my boys and the kids and moms I see as a nurse."

The profound understanding of this dynamic that had driven her life became the turning point of Nancy's work with me. Over the next few months, we explored further the way that her self-esteem was based solely on the care she provided for others. Slowly she came to see that even without hair or the energy to care for her husband and sons, she possessed value and worth. Sick as she was, she had every right to be attended to—and to feel good about deserving the attention. The change in Nancy was not a move toward selfishness or narcissism. Rather, by becoming more assertive about what she needed, Nancy became a more active participant in the treatment of her cancer and in the course of her life.

This change was not easy for Nancy to make. In the same way that the reality of cancer and chemotherapy had prompted the emotions typical to stress—anxiety and depression, for example—the change in her life brought up similar feelings. Still, Nancy discovered new resources within herself that allowed her to move toward a more active way of being in the world. The fighting spirit that Nancy was embracing now helped her in her struggle against the cancer. She also was better able to tolerate the uncertainty and lack of control that exist in cancer—and in the rest of life, for that matter. In addition, her emotional growth led to a more balanced relationship with her husband and children. Unclear at first whether he liked this "new" Nancy, her husband found over time that he felt better about himself when he knew more of what she needed. And her twin sons received an important lesson in altruism and compassion by doing their part to care for their mother while she was sick. Nancy even did better at work when she went back to nursing after recovering from the chemotherapy treatments. More attentive to her own needs and committed to articulating them, she built stronger relationships with the other nurses and the doctors, and found that now she rarely felt taken advantage of.

Cancer is a dark disorder with dark, emotional consequences. Like everyone who contracts the disease, Nancy suffered, in body and mind. At the same time, though, cancer is a bold light that illuminates the reality of life as a short-term lease, not a never-ending contract. So cancer can provide a catalyst for emotional growth. Nancy learned all these those lessons as she struggled to cope with her condition.

Although it has been five years since I saw Nancy, each holiday season she sends a card writing how well she is. There has been no recurrence of disease, her hair has grown back, and her energy has returned. Equally important, she has continued to live in the new way she learned when she was ill. Before cancer, Nancy tried to slip quietly through life. Then the disease shouted at her. She heard its call, and she grew. In learning how to cope with cancer, Nancy helped herself in the fight against the disease, and she gave herself a new lease on life. You can too. Let's figure out how, together.

2

COPING: WHAT WORKS, WHAT DOESN'T, AND WHY

NANCY'S STORY FROM CHAPTER 1 provides a classic look at the way a patient copes with cancer. Unfortunately, *cope* is a widely used word that, because of its very popularity, has lost much of its meaning. But for those of us who deal professionally with the emotional aspects of cancer, coping is a useful concept that helps explain much of what happens, both good and bad, as individuals go through their experience with the disease.

Coping occurs any time the outside world presents a challenge. That challenge—be it a mugger confronting you in an alley, or hearing the word *cancer* spoken when the results of a biopsy are reported to you—is a stressor. It is an external event that threatens some aspect of your existence. Your physical and emotional reactions to the stressor represent the stress you feel. In the case of the suddenly appearing mugger, those reactions add up to the classic physiology of the fight-or-flight response. Your blood pressure rises, your heart rate accelerates, your mouth goes dry and your palms moisten, your stomach and bowel turn queasy, and your muscles tense. You're physically prepared either to confront the threat or to run from it. Much the same happens in the case of cancer, although your response is far more complicated, both physically and emotionally, and it spans weeks, months, and years (rather than the seconds or minutes involved in a potential mugging).

Coping mechanisms refer to the conscious and unconscious ways a person adjusts to the stress of cancer without altering his or her goals. From another point of view, coping mechanisms are the ways individuals respond to life's stressors that prevent or control emotional distress and allow them to adapt to the reality of their situation. Cancer is an obvious source of emotional stress. The conscious and unconscious effort you mount to handle stress is the way you cope.

Consider what happened to Nancy when she first received a diagnosis of cancer of the bladder. Two of the coping mechanisms she adopted were denial and rationalization. In denial, she disavowed thoughts and feelings about the aspects of her new reality that she found intolerable on a conscious level. In rationalization, she justified, or argued herself out of, overwhelming external events. When Nancy told herself during sleepless nights, "Look, it's early stage. This is no big deal," she was both denying and rationalizing away her fears of having cancer. These coping mechanisms (which are called defenses and will be discussed in detail soon) are not conscious, willful choices, but unconscious reactions. For example, by focusing on the fact that hers was an early-stage cancer, Nancy initially treated the disease as nothing more serious than a bout of pneumonia—even if it did require abdominal surgery. Without considering what she was doing, Nancy downgraded or minimized the seriousness of her condition, acted as if little were wrong, and kept on going as usual. She adjusted to her sickness without changing any of her goals. She was still the wife, mother, and nurse she had always been; she continued to fulfill the roles that gave her life shape and meaning.

Nancy's personality style also played into her way of coping. She was a well-liked, flexible, and compliant person who relied too much on others to determine how well she dealt with her life, including cancer. It was only when the fatigue, hair loss, and nausea of chemotherapy increased Nancy's stressors to the breaking point, and made it increasingly difficult for her to serve as wife, mother, and nurse, that her personal coping style and ability to deny and rationalize came apart. Her basic emotional and physiological responses to the cancer now overwhelmed her, contributing to the sleeplessness, anxiety, and depression that brought her to me for treatment.

Antidepressant medication helped resolve Nancy's low moods, while psychotherapy sessions allowed her first to understand how she saw herself as valued only when she served others, then to build a new identity that accorded her value for being who she was. Over the course of Nancy's chemotherapy and her survivorship, these new coping mechanisms have proved to be viable, long-lasting, and beneficial. Denial and rationalization have become less central to how Nancy lives her life. In addition, Nancy has gained insight to those parts of her personality style that worked against her. She has been able to alter her way of being in the world—an emotional gain that has helped her cope more effectively.

Influences That Affect How Well You Cope

Four broad types of factors play into how a given individual copes with cancer. The first has to do with *the disease itself.* Where the cancer is located in the body, what stage it is in, and which treatment therapies have been proposed or are being implemented affect the magnitude of the stressor that cancer represents. For example, a woman who has been recently diagnosed with an in situ, or highly localized, cancer of the cervix has a much less serious disease, and less of a stressor to cope with, than does a woman who has been told that her cancer of the cervix has spread to distant organs and that, even with extensive and difficult surgery and other therapies, her odds for long-term survival are unfavorable.

Stage of life also plays into the effects that a particular kind of cancer has on the coping problem it presents. Even localized, in situ cervical cancer is likely to appear much more devastating to a young woman who has not yet had the children she wants than it does to a postmenopausal woman whose family is grown and living on their own.

The third set of factors has to do with *social support.* Scientists who have looked at the link between an individual's social network and the onset and outcome of illness have found that the more connected people are to family, faith communities, friends, and other groups, the better able they are to meet the challenge of serious disease. In fact, recent research has shown that being socially isolated may be as dangerous to your health as smoking.

Social support includes the comfort, assistance, and information an individual receives through formal or informal contacts with other individuals and groups. Support can take many forms and come from many sources. In Nancy's case, it was provided primarily by her husband and children, who never wavered in their concern and care for her, and by a couple of the nurses with whom she worked, who called or stopped by regularly while she was undergoing treatment. Ostensibly they were gossiping about goings-on in the clinic, but in fact they were keeping Nancy connected with a group that mattered to her, as well as showing their concern for her welfare. And since they were all medical professionals, Nancy was able to talk with them about aspects of her surgery and chemotherapy and enlist their aid in understanding what was happening to her body.

The forms of social support people seek out vary. Some people, especially men, may select more solitary avenues of support. They use chat rooms on the Internet, read recommended books about their illness, or simply spend time with their spouses, partners, or families. Others, especially women, flourish best when they seek out support groups, both formal and informal.

David Spiegel, M.D., and Catherine Classen, Ph. D., studied the value of group therapy sessions for women with advanced breast cancer. The women in these groups knew they were not alone in their experience, connected emotionally with others, asked for emotional support when they needed it, and provided it for others when it was requested. Instead of feeling alone and isolated in their suffering, they knew themselves to be part of a community. The results of this study showed that the symptoms of cancer were more controlled and there were more life-extending effects for women who were in the group therapy sessions.

Research also has shown consistently that simply sharing the experience of illness with someone helps an individual cope better with the disease. Often that role is filled by a spouse or another member of the nuclear family, but it can also involve an extended family member or a friend. This kind of emotional support may not only limit the psychological distress caused by the disease but possibly may help people live longer. In any event, it helps them live better because they cope more successfully, and more successful coping certainly improves quality of life (regardless of quantity).

The flip side of the connection between social support and coping is also true. A person with cancer who has no one to turn to, or a cancer patient who loses the support and help of someone close, suffers from additional distress. A friend, widowed suddenly while undergoing lumpectomy (removal of a cancerous mass) and radiation for breast cancer, said that her perceived abandonment by the man she thought she would spend the rest of her life with was more devastating to her than the disease itself.

Support, however, is by no means limited to the emotional variety. A young woman with small children and the diagnosis of cancer can benefit simply from a neighbor's offer to babysit a couple of afternoons a week, allowing her to get out of the house, walk in the park, or take in a movie. Enlightened medical professionals can provide important informational support when they tell cancer patients what to expect and help them to gain insight into the predictable course of their disease. For example, sometimes just knowing that a particular physical or emotional reaction to a type of surgery is normal can help resolve emotional distress and enhance the patient's ability to cope with the cancer treatment.

The fourth set of factors that influence coping has to do with the *resources, values, and emotional patterns of the individual.* Some of these factors are obvious. Personal and cognitive skills play a role. Children have a much more limited repertoire of coping mechanisms than do adults, and they are more vulnerable to, and less defended against, the stresses caused by the disease. Typically, the more psychologically mature one is, the more resources that person has to draw on for coping.

Previous personal experiences with cancer greatly affect coping. A person who has watched a parent or sibling suffer from a lengthy illness is more likely to adopt an attitude of hopelessness than is someone with a similar cancer who has seen a family member go into remission and live well for years.

Religion, spirituality, and belief in an afterlife also play a role. Some people suffer from a deeply ingrained feeling that cancer is a punishment for sin, whereas others see their suffering as a necessary path to a higher plane of existence and accept their disease as part of a divine plan. And there are those who are influenced by the moral code of their religion irrespective of any belief in an afterlife. For example, the Judeo-Christian ethic emphasizes selflessness and the stoic acceptance of suffering. These are worthy moral precepts, but they can be carried to an extreme that makes it difficult for a cancer patient to complain appropriately about pain and to act like a sick person deserving of care.

Other personal factors are so complex and extensive in their effect that we will take a closer look at two of them: the individual's personality, and the meaning that he or she attaches to cancer because of his or her emotional history.

How Personality Type Affects Coping

Personality refers to the characteristic ways that a person thinks, feels, and behaves. It is the overall, ingrained, emotional and behavioral pattern that evolves, both consciously and unconsciously, as an individual progresses through life and meets the various challenges and opportunities offered by his or her environment. Personality traits are the various components that make up the personality. Sometimes, the sum of an individual's personality traits is referred to as his or her *character*.

Personality traits are so key to a person's way of being that we usually take them for granted. In fact, we are most likely to notice them only when someone we know well displays a trait not usually associated with that person. Nancy is a good example (see Chapter 1). When she first began asserting her own needs, her husband was startled. He actually said to her, "This isn't like you." And he was right: Nancy's self-promotion ran counter to the character she had previously displayed. She was changing her style and behaving out of character.

That phrase points to something that psychiatrists, psychologists, and other students of human behavior have long noted: People can be grouped into elementary personality types based on their dominant traits. If you have a sense of your own or your loved one's personality type, you have some ability to predict how the stress of cancer will make itself known and how the individual is likely to respond. So let's examine these basic personality types so that you have a grasp on how you or a loved one may tend to respond to a diagnosis of cancer.

But as we work through the description of personality types, keep a number of facts in mind. First, *no one fits any single category perfectly.* In fact, while one type tends to predominate in each of us, we may well exhibit important traits from other personality types as well. Individuals are, after all, individual, and each one of us represents a unique blend of traits. In their most extreme and rigid forms, each personality type explained in this section (with the exception of the adaptive) may be viewed as a disorder, but in their more usual, milder expressions, they are collections of particular strengths and weaknesses that both contribute to and detract from our ability to cope. Second, *personalities are the product of early learning and genetics,* and not conscious creations of the individuals who have them. As research has probed more and more deeply into the chemical components of personality, it has been suggested that a part of how we think, feel, and behave may be inherited. Third, and unfortunately, *the names attached to many of the personality types often carry pejorative meanings.* When Sigmund Freud first used the term *anal,* he had a specific developmental meaning in mind. Today the word has entered common parlance as a put-down for anyone seen as rigid and precise. Understand that the names given to each personality type arise from long-used scientific jargon and are not moral judgments. To avoid the pejorative connotations that stick to many of the standard psychiatric labels, I have changed the usual names to more commonplace ones (although I have mentioned the usual scientific label in the explanatory text that follows).

Adaptive Personality

The *adaptive* personality type is emotionally mature and evolved. Such individuals have a solid self-esteem and realistic expectations of their world. These people are well liked, pleasant, and neither overly needy nor demanding. They tend to be open, empathic, and able to tolerate frustration. In addition, their positive interpersonal skills lead to intimate relationships and a large support group.

Cancer is a significant stressor, so adaptive types have appropriate anxiety and depression. But this is brief. The disease is then taken up as a challenge with flexibility, insight, and optimism.

Such people usually cope extremely well with cancer. Their character equips them to deal with the rigors of diagnosis, treatment, and survivorship.

Dependent Personality

This set of traits reveals itself in actions that often appear needy and naive. *Dependent* people are overly reliant on others for their emotional gratification, and they often respond with anxiety and fear to situations that require them to be independent. At the same time, dependent people can be generous and attentive.

Serious illness poses a major dilemma for people with dependent personalities. They have a wish for boundless care and often appear highly demanding, yet they are driven by the fear that the people they most depend on will abandon them. An illness such as cancer, which requires long-term treatment and necessitates prolonged contact with caregivers such as physicians, nurses, and hospice workers, poses a particular challenge for the dependent personality. People with this set of traits respond best to directions and demands that are gentle and firm but not critical. More than anything else, they need to know that they will not be abandoned and that their needs for care will be met.

Control-Oriented Personality

Also known as *obsessive-compulsive,* such individuals tend to be emotionally reserved, rational and logical, systematic and orderly, and sometimes unbending or even rigid. They often focus on the letter of the law more than the spirit and pay close attention to minute details, sometimes at the cost of missing the big picture. Control-oriented individuals tend to be conscientious, concerned with issues of right and wrong, frugal, and self-disciplined.

Psychodynamic theory suggests that these personality traits, in part, develop as a way of controlling aggression. Cancer threatens the self-control explicit in this psychological structure. These people tend to become more rigid in response to the disease and to seek information about their condition from physicians, libraries, the Internet, and other sources. Sometimes, because they desperately wish to remain in control of their situation, they have trouble making up their minds about key issues such as treatment options. They respond best to careful, methodical instructions and detailed information, and, to the extent possible, they like to participate in and have control over their own care. Control-oriented individuals can be focused, goal-oriented, extremely responsible and dependable—traits that make them conscientious patients who follow their treatment regimens rigorously.

Overemotional Personality

Also called *histrionic,* a word that comes from a Latin word meaning "actor," overemotional people have an actor's flair for drama and displays of feeling. They are full of panache and style, are often larger than life, and are given to display and dramatization. Characteristically, histrionic people are charming, charismatic, imaginative, entertaining, and often seductive. Sometimes they have a powerful need to be admired, and they often seek reassurance that they are indeed attractive enough to be worthy of that admiration. Cancer poses a powerful challenge to this self-image. Histrionic men fear a diminution of physical prowess and power, and women are threatened by the possible loss of physical beauty. Flattery is a strong motivator for histrionic people, and it can help them follow their treatment regimen.

Self-Centered Personality

Self-centered people are also called *narcissistic,* a word that comes from an ancient myth told in its best-known form by the classical Roman poet,

Ovid. Narcissus was a beautiful young man who fell in love with his own image reflected in a pool of water, tried to embrace himself, and drowned. Self-centered individuals are like histrionic people in their flair for drama and display, but they focus more on themselves than on their audience. They love being the most important individuals in each and every setting in which they find themselves, and they have a way of occupying center stage no matter where they are. At its best, the narcissistic personality is charismatic, dramatically entertaining, and highly creative, but it can also come across as arrogant, smug, and vain.

Narcissistic people want to be perceived as perfect, and cancer makes them feel decidedly imperfect. They also see the cancer as occupying center stage—the place *they* prefer to occupy. They want to be cared for by the very best physicians at the very best clinics, and they want to do better on their therapeutic regimen than any patient has done before.

Guarded Personality

People with guarded, or *paranoid,* personality traits are often suspicious or querulous, and they find it difficult to trust others. Since guarded individuals usually think the worst of the people around them, they feel most comfortable in situations they control. They tend to be fearful and highly sensitive to criticisms or slights, which they perceive as attacks directed against them. Cancer is perceived as just one more attack. By the same token, guarded individuals tend to be highly methodical in how they work out solutions to problems, which can be a strength during cancer treatment. Guarded people sometimes become mistrustful of physicians and other caregivers ("I don't think he's doing everything for me that he could be doing"), and they often have trouble submitting to invasive procedures such as biopsies or the placement of a shunt for chemotherapy.

Isolated Personality

The isolated, or *schizoid,* personality tends to be withdrawn and aloof at times, even eccentric. Sometimes people with this group of traits are reclusive, remote, reserved, and unlikely to involve themselves in social activities. It is thought that people with isolated traits keep their distance as a way of maintaining their internal psychological balance. They fear intrusion, which cancer serves up in a big way. To avoid this threat, isolated people may deny their illness or minimize its seriousness. Above all else, such people need reassurance that their privacy and integrity will be respected throughout treatment. The most striking strength of the isolated personality is its ability to perceive and think in unusual and interesting ways. Because isolated people are more lone wolves than cattle in the herd, they often see the dilemmas, challenges, and issues of cancer treatment in an atypical, idiosyncratic light.

Avoidant Personality

People with an *avoidant* personality want everything to go smoothly, hate confrontation, and retreat from distasteful situations. In a way, the avoidant person is like the ostrich of myth: if the big bird just buries its head in the sand, the lion will go away. Cancer, of course, is one big hungry lion, and the avoidant person tries to steer clear of the disease and its anxiety by failing to follow through. Anxiety keeps avoidant people from seeking medical care in general, and when they notice a problem that could indicate cancer, such as a lump in the breast or blood in the urine, they are likely to postpone going to the doctor, leading to a delay in diagnosis. Avoidant people often don't show up for chemotherapy sessions, doctor's visits, periodic bone scans, and the like. They sit and worry about their predicament instead of facing its reality by adhering to their treatment or diagnostic regimen. The good side of the avoidant personality is that it makes people easy and pleasant to be with. Since avoidant people dislike confrontation, they make few demands.

Self-Defeating Personality

Also referred to as *masochistic,* self-defeating people have low self-esteem and a lot of guilt. They often unconsciously create situations that lead them to failure. They tend to see cancer as a deserved punishment and to assume that the disease will get them in the end no matter what they do. Self-defeating people are self-effacing, and, when that trait is coupled with a good sense of humor, they can be funny and entertaining.

How Emotional History Affects
the Meaning of Cancer

Cancer is not simply a disease of the body. It is a serious illness that carries a unique psychological import for each personality type. Where the self-centered person sees cancer as a challenge to his or her ability to occupy center stage, the isolated person views the disease as an invasion of a closely held and highly prized privacy. Cancer is different things to different people.

The meaning of the disease varies not only with personality type but also with an individual's emotional history. Who, what, and where we have been in life is central to cancer's import, as these case histories show.

A Sense of Guilt Can Play a Part

Jack, a successful fifty-five-year-old insurance broker, was outgoing and upbeat. He enjoyed his buddies as much as his wife and children. The captain of his high school football team and the "most likely to succeed" graduate of the local community college, Jack always mixed pleasure with work. Unfortunately, one early pleasure, cigarette smoking, grew into a two-pack-a-day habit that, despite several halfhearted attempts to quit, Jack could never quite drop.

Over the prior year, Jack had suffered repeated bouts of bronchitis, and he noticed that he ran out of breath easily while playing golf. Secretly worried about a link between his smoking and his respiratory problems, Jack went to see his doctor. An extensive work-up confirmed his worst fears: lung cancer.

That was the bad news. The good news was that Jack had a relatively early stage of a type of lung cancer that responds well to aggressive chemotherapy. The treatment wouldn't be easy, but it offered distinct hope for controlling the disease. Given Jack's upbeat nature and strong macho streak, one would have expected him to meet the cancer head-on, ready to fight. Instead, Jack sat restlessly in the oncologist's examining room, rubbing his hands together and experiencing heart palpitations and sweaty palms. Then he told the oncologist he was refusing chemotherapy.

"I don't want any poisons put in me," Jack said. "In fact, I don't want any treatment at all."

The oncologist, who had known Jack socially ever since they had been students in high school together, was stunned. "But, Jack, there's every reason to think this will work. Why are you saying no?"

Jack snapped, "Doc, this is really none of your business. Quite frankly, I don't even deserve to get well."

"Why not?" the doctor asked.

"Well, this is my own fault, damn it! Everyone knows smoking causes cancer. This disease must be my punishment."

Guilt can be a common reaction to cancer. Regret over lifestyle and habits, often superimposed on rigid familial and religious upbringing, often leads to excessive distress and belief that the disease is a retribution or retaliation for some past wrong.

Fortunately, psychotherapy with a psychiatrist helped Jack understand the sources of his feelings so that he could come to grips with his guilt. He was the last son of parents who were committed to using their children in their own ambitious climb up the social ladder. Whenever Jack succeeded—for example, when he was named football captain—his parents lavished him with love and attention. But when he did something wrong—for instance, when he received less than stellar grades—they scolded or teased him mercilessly, or sometimes ignored him altogether, as if he had ceased to exist. Thus, Jack had come to believe that he was morally responsible for each and every event in his life, particularly his failures. This background was reinforced by Jack's fundamentalist church, which lived to denounce sin and exhaled the hot fumes of fire and brimstone. No wonder Jack saw his cancer as a punishment! As Jack came to understand how his parents had shaped him, and as he opened himself to the merciful and loving part of his God, Jack regained his typical optimistic fighting spirit and agreed to treatment, which was successful. He also finally quit smoking. Jack returned to a full life of work and play and many years of remission—without cigarettes.

Many cancer patients, even those who do not come from a fundamentalist background, find themselves in a similar emotional situation.

Everyone's personality contains the part that Sigmund Freud called the *superego,* where rules, regulations, and moral and ethical codes are internalized. The superego comes into play when we judge ourselves. In cancer, with its anxiety and depression, self-judgment often becomes unnecessarily harsh, quickly growing into an ongoing source of guilt.

Our Psychological and Biological Predisposition Makes an Impact

Tom, a single twenty-eight-year-old salesman originally from Los Angeles, lived alone in a New York City apartment. Like most young men, he took his good health for granted until several days of extreme fatigue accompanied by fever and chills sent him to the emergency room of the local hospital. A complete blood count—a routine test for such symptoms—revealed a markedly elevated number of white blood cells, many of which were atypical. A pathologist and a hematologist studied the blood samples and came to the same disturbing diagnosis of acute leukemia.

Tom's response to the bad news was typical. For several days, he alternated between shock, denial, and disbelief, then entered a couple of weeks of transient anxiety, sleeplessness, and late-night existential musings about the value and meaning of life. After that, he returned to his usual style, which was even, quiet, and friendly. Meanwhile, he consulted with a number of specialists about his treatment options and shared the information over the telephone with his family back in California.

About four weeks after Tom's diagnosis, his co-workers noticed a marked change in his personality. Tom was now the first to show up for work in the morning and the last to leave at night. His energy was boundless, his enthusiasm unmatched. He spoke rapidly, loudly, and tangentially, and there was a new note of boasting and grandiosity in the way he talked to colleagues and customers. Even worse, he didn't know when to stop talking.

At about the same time, Tom's next-door neighbor complained to the landlord about the sudden rise in the volume of Tom's stereo and his loud, off-key sing-alongs. When the landlord asked Tom to turn it down, Tom verbally attacked the man. The barrage was so hostile and threatening that the landlord called Tom's brother, who immediately flew to New York.

Tom had been hospitalized twice in his late teens: the first time for a suicidal depression, the second for a severe manic episode. Diagnosed with bipolar disorder—also known as manic depression, an emotional disorder characterized by dramatic mood swings—Tom was put on a regimen of lithium (a mood stabilizer) and received supportive psychotherapy. After moving to New York City, Tom continued to take the medication under prescription from a local internist. But when Tom received the news that he had leukemia, he stopped the lithium because of an unfounded fear that the medication was the cause of his cancer.

Tom's brother convinced him to talk with a psychiatrist, and that was how he came to me. He agreed to go back on his medication. He and I then worked together with his oncologist to help keep his moods stable as he moved into the rigors and demands of bone marrow transplant therapy.

Tom's experience is a strong reminder of the fact that every person has an inherent biological and psychological predisposition, providing both strengths and weaknesses. Because of the severe stress it causes, cancer has a way of exposing and exploiting these Achilles' heels in our individual makeup. These predispositions are important to understand in cancer patients.

The Value We Place on Life Becomes Clear

In most people, cancer creates a powerful anxiety, because it threatens a deep-seated desire to live. But every now and then, an individual's life experiences can prompt an opposite response.

Julie was a fine arts graduate student in her mid-twenties who had come from Paris for evaluation. Her well-to-do father had set up the consultation at Sloan-Kettering after doctors in France were divided in their opinion as to whether cancer was causing Julie's ongoing stomach problems. After Julie arrived in New York, diagnostic tests revealed that she had a very rare type of stomach cancer. Fortunately, this particular type of cancer has little tendency to metastasize. Although the surgery to remove it was difficult, the entire tumor was excised. As far as Julie's surgeon was concerned, she was completely cured.

Yet this momentously good news had a shocking effect on Julie. Instead of experiencing elation at her release from a possible death sentence, Julie became highly anxious and depressed. Another psychiatrist had interviewed her only the day before, trying to get at the root of her emotional condition, but she told him nothing except that she wanted antianxiety medication. Julie was withdrawn and uncooperative, and her doctor had no idea what to try next to find out what was going on with her.

Hoping that a fresh face might prompt a different response, I went to Julie's private room and introduced myself. She was a classically beautiful young woman, petite and delicate, her angelic face surrounded by long black hair. When I asked if I could talk with her for a bit, Julie agreed.

For perhaps ten minutes we spoke politely and quietly as I asked mundane questions and she gave fittingly ordinary answers. Then, without warning, Julie bolted upright in bed, and declared loudly, "This is all absurd!"

"Absurd?" I asked. "What's absurd?"

"This is all absurd!" she shouted again with even more energy. She repeated the word *absurd* dozens of times.

In the next few minutes, anger turned to sadness, and her eyes filled with tears. I simply sat quietly, letting the emotions wash through. Then she said, "They cut out the door that would have let me escape from this life."

Her metaphor stunned me. Was cancer the door she meant? Had she wanted to die from cancer as a way of escaping a life she couldn't stand? I asked Julie to tell me more.

As far as Julie could reach back into her memory, she had fantasized about dying. These fantasies weren't nightmares; rather, they were dreams of relief and escape. She had flirted with suicide since early childhood, making one gentle gesture at self-destruction after another. She had the desire for death but not enough will to succeed at killing herself.

"But why?" I asked. "Why would someone with so much to live for want to die?"

She answered, "My father has always treated me like a toy. He dominates everything I do. He cares only about my outward appearance. He is a big shot, and I am his showpiece. For the rest, I do not count."

Julie had no inner sense of who she was, and she felt empty. Eager to escape this nonexistence, she had seized upon cancer as an ideal way out.

"A young woman dying of cancer—that is noble. Cancer gave me an acceptable reason to die," Julie explained. "It made people feel sorry for me, and they gave me their love. And I didn't have to go on living like this."

Then cancer played a dirty trick on Julie: It let her live. She responded with an angry despair at having been robbed of an ideal opportunity to escape a life she had never found livable and whose prospects seemed horrible. Ironically, good news about cancer had deprived her of the death fantasy she found familiar and comfortable. No longer able to escape from the reality of her life by imagining an imminent death, Julie now had the seed from which to grow a new life—one that might hold meaning for her.

Since most people want life, they find cancer a terrible source of anxiety because it threatens them with death. Julie's response was just the opposite. She had a desire for death as an escape, and, when cancer's convenient exit was removed and she found life staring her in the face, anxiety about an uncertain and intolerable future overwhelmed her. Few people find themselves in Julie's shoes. Yet Julie's case, in its strange reversed way, shows how deeply cancer strikes at our core of emotional meaning.

Additional Factors That Impact the Ability to Cope

Guilt, personal and biological disposition, and your personal relationship to the issues of life and death are not the only things that affect how well you cope. A number of other medical, social, and psychological factors can add to the difficulty of coping by making you more vulnerable to distress.

Medical Factors

- *More physical symptoms.* A cancer that is obvious in its manifestations, such as a brain tumor that is causing problems with memory, speech, and coordination, is more of a stressor than is a "silent" tumor such as prostate cancer or a small breast lump. The pain, fatigue, nausea, and other effects of the cancer and the treatment increase the stressors.
- *More advanced cancer at diagnosis.* The further along the cancer is and the lesser likelihood of successful treatment, the more of a stressor it poses, and the more difficult the coping task.
- *Poor relationship with the physician.* Individuals who don't trust their doctors or feel good about their care experience more distress.
- *Short-time survival prospects after the diagnosis.* Some cancers, such as lung or pancreatic cancer, move very rapidly and confront the individual with the probability of death more quickly. Obviously, this increases the challenge to cope.

Social Factors

- *Lower socioeconomic status.* People who lack good sick leave benefits, adequate health insurance, and a healthy savings account are going to find the disruption of cancer more stressful than those individuals fortunate enough to have good insurance, plenty of accumulated sick leave, and money in the bank.
- *Marital and family problems.* Cancer can add difficulty to even the best marriage. In a relationship marred by conflict, abuse, or poor communication, cancer simply adds to the problems. In addition, partners with the disease are deprived of an important source of solace and support if they are not getting along well with their spouse or significant other. Likewise, acting-out, needy, immature children, siblings, or parents add to the cancer patient's burden and make coping more difficult.
- *Poor social support network.* People who expect little support from others, don't ask for such help, and isolate themselves feel more distress during the crises of cancer than do those who assume that others will

help, ask for assistance when they need it, and are connected to faith communities, interest groups, extended families, friends, and other support networks.

Psychological Factors

- *History of psychiatric problems.* As we have discussed in this chapter in the cases of Tom and Julie, cancer has a way of worsening existing mental health problems.
- *High anxiety.* Some people are particularly prone to anxiety, even under good circumstances. Cancer makes the anxiety worse.
- *Low ego strength.* Ego strength refers to a person's emotional assets, such as flexibility, empathy, and a sense of humor. People with high ego strength are mature and adaptable; those with low ego strength are immature and inflexible. The more psychologically healthy an individual is, the better able he or she is to meet cancer's challenge. People who lack maturity find this task all the more daunting.
- *High degree of denial.* People who excessively deny or falsely minimize the seriousness of their condition are more likely to suffer from depression or anxiety as underlying fears break through their defense mechanisms. Although it may seem initially more frightening, facing up to the reality of cancer—to the extent that the individual is psychologically capable—builds a better foundation in the long term for coping.
- *More concerns of all kinds.* A young single working mom with an ex-husband who is a deadbeat dad is going to find cancer far more of a crisis than an older woman whose children are grown and gone, whose marriage is strong, and whose finances are secure. Cancer adds another burden to an already heavy load.
- *A sense of surrender.* Lacking fighting spirit has been shown to increase the level of distress people feel as they face cancer. In contrast, the sense of engaging the disease as an opponent, instead of surrendering to it, mobilizes psychological resources and helps the patient deal with the distress of each cancer crisis. Alternating between hopelessness and helplessness or bearing up without complaint and exhibiting extreme stoicism are not useful.

- *Alcohol and drug abuse.* Because they serve to mask and suppress feelings—which have a way of emerging anyway—alcohol and other drugs only heighten distress over the long term.
- *Poor coping strategies.* Some people cope less effectively than others, partly as a result of personality style, and partly because they have never learned better ways to deal with challenges.

Typical Defense Mechanisms

Cancer challenges who we are. It can threaten the very existence of life itself, and even early-stage localized cancers force one to recognize mortality. Equally important, cancer changes the psychological perception of the self. In a way, the disease says that you are no longer who you once were. The self doesn't like this; it wants to protect its identity by holding on. Protecting one's identity is the function of the coping strategies known as *defense mechanisms*—the unconscious processes that operate within the psyche outside of one's awareness. They are not the result of willful, conscious decision, and they serve to provide relief from emotional conflict and anxiety. Our fundamental defense mechanisms are:

- *Denial.* The individual disavows thoughts, feelings, wishes, needs, or aspects of the outside world that are intolerable to the conscious mind. Nancy provides an excellent example (see Chapter 1). When her cancer was diagnosed, she denied the level of threat it posed to her. Another common example of denial is someone ignoring a suspicious lump or mole instead of seeking medical attention.
- *Displacement.* Emotions, ideas, or wishes are transferred from their original object to a substitute that is more acceptable. A cancer patient who comes home angry from a difficult session with the physician may dump that anger on his or her children or spouse.
- *Projection.* Emotionally unacceptable ideas and feelings in the self are attributed to someone else. A person who fears that he or she is dying of cancer but who cannot accept this reality consciously may say, "You know, that doctor of mine thinks I'm going to die."
- *Rationalization.* The individual makes intolerable feelings, actions, or

motives tolerable by giving them a plausible and acceptable motive. A person who wants to stop chemotherapy in the middle of treatment because of its unpleasant side effects might say, "You know, this cancer isn't as bad as they tell me. It won't make any difference if I stop now." Since the full course of chemotherapy has to be completed for the treatment to be successful, the patient is engaging in rationalization that is emotionally and physically unhealthy.

- *Reaction formation.* It defends the self by adopting ideas, attitudes, and actions that are the opposite of unacceptable impulses harbored unconsciously within the self. A patient who is irritated by her oncologist's arrogant, know-it-all manner might bring the physician expensive gifts as apparent tokens of respect. Or another patient who feels angry at the nurse who administers the chemotherapy that leaves him feeling sick and weak for days afterward may find himself falling inexplicably in love with her.

- *Regression.* The individual slips back into infantile or childlike patterns of reacting and thinking. An older child who is diagnosed with leukemia and begins wetting the bed is regressing.

- *Sublimation.* Unacceptable drives are diverted into channels that are personally and socially acceptable. An artist I know who contracted breast cancer expressed her fear of the disease by painting her self-portrait—bald from the effects of chemotherapy—next to an oversized, lurking vulture. The painting gave her a sense of peace because it expressed feelings she could not otherwise find a way of dealing with. Sublimation is a particularly healthy defense mechanism.

Assessing the Effectiveness of Our Defense Mechanisms

Personality types and defense mechanisms embody a fascinating psychological paradox. On the one hand, they are undeniable and extremely important aspects of maintaining the psychological equilibrium necessary to effective coping. On the other, they can get in the way by maintaining a false sense of security and making effective coping impossible.

Once again, Nancy offers a good example (see Chapter 1). During diagnosis and surgical treatment, she used denial to protect herself against the reality of the disease. Denial can be an effective and useful coping strategy. We all do it to one extent or another, and I doubt that any of us could get through an ordinary day unless we repeatedly and unconsciously utilized denial. Without some level of denial, the world's repeated injustices and widespread suffering would overwhelm almost all of us. It lets us block out some conflicts, pains, and injustices and focus on others. In Nancy's case, denial helped her tolerate surgery and retain her psychological balance. This was something Nancy was used to doing; for years, she had denied her own needs. Denying her fears about cancer was just more of the same.

But then, under the rigors of chemotherapy, her denial lost its efficacy. The feelings Nancy was trying to hide—fear and anxiety about death, extended sickness, the loss of personal control, and her lack of self-worth when she was unable to function as a wife, mother, and nurse—broke through her defense mechanism. What had been an effective coping strategy was no longer working. Her depression signaled that a change was in order. Nancy needed to take a hard look at her psychological history and learn new ways to cope with the demands of cancer and life.

The same paradox holds true of personality traits. When a person is able to make use of the strengths and weaknesses represented by his or her character in a way that contributes to psychological equilibrium, then all is well. But if the personality type turns into a rigid, inflexible posture, then it leaves the individual poorly equipped to cope effectively and the person can even develop the kind of cancer-related psychological disorders we will look at in Chapter 7.

Two former cancer patients, Max and Sam, serve as excellent examples. There were many similarities between these two men. Both were unmarried and without children, in their late thirties, involved in computer-related jobs, distinctly obsessive or control-oriented in their personality styles, and diagnosed with non-Hodgkin's lymphoma, a cancer of the lymphatic system.

Max enjoyed his solitude, but he wasn't a loner; rather, he chose his friends carefully. Max was intensely enthusiastic about science and rock-and-roll. He read science books voraciously, collected tapes and CDs with a passion, and could chitchat the history of rock-and-roll in such detail that you'd think he was a staffer at *Rolling Stone* rather than a systems engineer. When Max learned he had cancer, he faced the disease intellectually—that is, he spent hours in the local library and on the Internet, and in a matter of weeks he knew so much about non-Hodgkin's lymphoma that his oncologist jokingly suggested that Max come in as a consultant on some of the more difficult cases.

Max did experience the usual bouts of transient anxiety and insomnia, particularly early in his diagnosis and treatment, but he overcame them by achieving a kind of intellectual mastery over the disease. He was also adept at focused denial. He learned that his specific type of lymphoma often goes into long periods of remission, but sometimes proves life-threatening nonetheless. He blocked that last fact from his mind, focused on achieving a remission and went about his treatment and the rest of his life with considerable energy. Clearly, his coping style was effective.

Sam preferred science fiction to science, and his musical preference tended more to Bach than the Beatles, yet his personality style was similar to Max's. When he discovered he had cancer, he also tackled the disease intellectually. At first, he seemed well balanced psychologically, despite the expected insomnia and anxiety. Then a few weeks after his diagnosis, things began to unravel. Sam had learned an enormous amount about his disease, but he couldn't make up his mind about the treatment options. He agonized over every detail, slipped into a mood that spiraled downward, lost his desire to eat, and sat around the house with too little energy to even turn on the TV and watch a ballgame. Sam's sister, a social worker, recognized that he was heading toward a major depression and talked about this with Sam's oncologist. Alerted to Sam's declining mood, the physician then suggested that Sam consult with a psychiatrist. Psychotherapy and medication halted the depression and enabled Sam to put together a more effective coping style.

I suspect that the difference in Sam and Max lay in their psychological histories. Max was a well-loved child who received a strong sense of his inherent self-worth from his family. Sam came from a colder, neglectful background, where he was forced to spend a great deal of time alone, and he didn't trust himself to make good friends. Still, the important point is that Max's coping strategy worked for him, helping him maintain an even mental keel as he entered treatment. In Sam's case, his coping strategy collapsed as the primitive feelings of fear and anxiety broke through.

There is no single right way of coping. Rather, each individual has to find the style that works for him or her.

How Well Am I Coping?

A coping strategy is effective for you if it accomplishes these goals:

- Holds your distress to a tolerable level
- Helps you maintain your self-worth
- Supports the establishment or continuation of good relationships with your spouse, children, co-workers, companions, lover, friends, and/or other significant people in your life
- Helps you recover your physical functions
- Makes it more likely that you will be in a beneficial situation after physical recovery—that is, you'll be able to live your life with a sense of meaning and purpose

If a coping strategy is working for you, follow it. And if it doesn't, then it is time to seek out new ways of dealing with your cancer. Let's look closely at some of these ways.

The Many Ways to Cope Heathfully

The anxiety and depression that surround cancer rest on a fundamental dilemma: The problem you face now exceeds your ability to deal with it. It's something like standing on a beach and watching the leading edge of a tidal wave about to break over you. Even if you know how to swim, it's a lot more water than you've ever had to deal with before.

Still, there *are* skills you can learn and resources you can call on as needed. This section lists the basic coping modalities, both informal and formal. We will explore them, particularly the formal modalities, in greater detail as we look further into the psychology of cancer's course in the following chapters.

Informal Ways of Coping

- *Religion and spirituality.* Prayer works—and it doesn't really matter what kind of prayer it is: Christian, Jewish, Muslim, Hindu, Buddhist, or whatever. What counts more than the content or language of the prayer is the ritual of placing trust in a reality greater than oneself. The structure and support of a formal religion, or some sense of spirituality, create an environment conducive to peace and personal growth. Many people find great solace in seeking a meaningful exploration of life and what may exist beyond.
- *Exercise.* Working out helps, but avoid short, fierce bursts of activity (even if you feel up to it) such as running wind sprints in the outfield. Such activity increases the breathing rate precipitously and causes chemical changes that can add to feelings of anxiety. Instead, focus on exercise that raises heart and breathing rates moderately for an extended period of time. A number of options are available, among them jogging, walking, bicycling, training in a weight room, aerobics, and swimming. This kind of exercise contributes to overall health and wellness, and it helps lower blood pressure and heart rate, thus controlling some of the manifestations of anxiety. Exercise also increases physical mastery, an important feeling at a time when the body often acts as if it is very much out of control. Finally, exercise induces the release of certain brain chemicals that increase feelings of well-being and reduce the physiological reactions underlying anxiety.
- *Massage and other tactile modalities.* Massage, a form of therapeutic touch, is useful for coping. Humans draw strength from physical connections, be it a mother soothing an infant or lovers holding hands at a rock concert. Massage also helps relax muscles tightened by anxiety. Also, aromatherapy (use of various oils and fragrances to bring about

relaxation) and acupressure (an Eastern medical practice similar to acupuncture where pressure is applied to certain areas instead of inserting needles) appear to have a similar beneficial effect.

- *Travel.* Most people feel better when they change their circumstances. Take yourself to a place you like, even if it's only a short distance away, and you may discover both better clarity about the problems you face and more strength to face them.
- *Entertainment and art.* Laughing helps, a point made most eloquently in Norman Cousins's *Anatomy of an Illness.* Cousins argued that humor, smiling, and laughter all aided his recovery from a life-threatening illness. Music of any sort that interests you, painting, sculpting, theater, reading, writing, and other modes of aesthetic enjoyment are rewarding ways to take a break from illness.

Formal Modalities

- *Support groups.* Fortunately, there are many kinds of support groups that can help you come to terms with the difficult issues raised by cancer. Some include people with different kinds of cancer, whereas others include only those with a given type of disease, such as cancer of the breast or colon. Some admit people of only one gender; others welcome males and females. Some accept patients and their partners; others, only patients, partners, or family members. Various settings for these groups are possible, such as the general community, a hospital, or a health care organization. The type of group that works best for you is determined by your specific disease and your psychological needs. You may try more than one before you find the one that best suits you. Please see the Resources section at the end of this book for more information on finding support groups.
- *Psychotherapy.* This approach entails a talking treatment using psychological techniques to relieve emotional problems. As we will discuss in much more detail in later chapters, turning to a professional for help is a fine way to cope, not a sign of weakness or character flaw. Therapy can be conducted for the individual, within a group setting, or inside a family. And there are a variety of treatments to choose from, ranging

from longer-term psychodynamic therapy to shorter-term, crisis-focused modalities (see Chapter 7).

- *Relaxation techniques.* There are two basic types. The first, called progressive muscle relaxation, is drawn from behavior therapy. You lie in a quiet place with your arms at your side and you alternately tense and relax each group of muscles, working upward from toes to head. The second, developed by Harvard cardiologist Herbert Benson and widely publicized through his book *The Relaxation Response,* holds that the body has an innate relaxation mechanism that is the opposite of the usual fight-or-flight response. This relaxation response can be induced by sitting in a quiet place for ten to twenty minutes, focusing the mind on the breath or a single repeated word, and disregarding distracting thoughts by returning quietly and without judgment to breath or word. Relaxation techniques lower heart and breathing rate, decrease oxygen consumption, and reduce the levels of chemicals in the blood that rise in response to stress.

- *Meditation.* Again, there are two main types. The passive approaches achieve relaxation by passively disregarding intrusive thoughts. Active approaches, sometimes called mindful meditation and exemplified by the work of Jon Kabat-Zinn and Zen master Thich Nhat Hanh, seek to achieve a new perspective on the experience of sensations by focusing on specific thoughts and feelings. Learning to meditate is an excellent antidote to the anxiety that accompanies every crisis in cancer. Meditation comes in a variety of flavors, such as Zen, Vipassana, Tibetan, Christian (e.g., Roman Catholic monastic or Quaker), and Jewish (e.g., davening in prayer). All of them work, and all, though different in their specifics, share a common core: focused concentration and heightened relaxation. The value of meditation for people with cancer is that it teaches relaxation at a time when the outside world may be frightening and upsetting. By lowering heart and breathing rates and bringing mental focus to a single point, meditation calms the body and the mind.

For people with panic disorder—one of the mental illnesses that appears in a small percentage of people with cancer (see Chapter 6)—meditation can be problematic, however. Most forms of meditation focus on controlling breathing, which, in someone with panic disorder, can be so frightening that a panic attack may ensue. The solution is to learn a meditation technique that focuses on a process other than breathing from a practitioner who understands panic disorder.

In general, it is better to learn meditation from an individual teacher rather than a book or audiotape. Many counselors and psychotherapists are trained in meditation or can recommend a teacher.

- *Medical hypnosis.* Despite the nightclub hucksterism surrounding hypnosis, scientific data suggest that it may be useful in alleviating anxiety. Hypnosis produces an unusual psychological state. Most of the time, extreme concentration is accompanied by a high level of arousal. Under hypnosis, you are both very relaxed and very focused, a state that leaves you open to new ways of thinking and feeling. A therapist can teach you self-hypnosis as a way of relaxing, particularly in anticipation of unpleasant events such as biopsies and chemotherapy sessions. Indeed, hypnosis is particularly good against anticipatory anxiety—that sense of fear that arises when you think ahead to the unpleasant event. It is also an excellent adjunct to pain management.
- *Psychotropic medications.* As we will discuss in detail, psychiatrists have at their disposal an impressive array of drugs that are effective against depression and anxiety in all its many forms. Used in conjunction with psychotherapy, support groups, and other coping modalities, medication can help normalize mood and make it easier to face the current cancer crisis. The types of medications that are often prescribed are discussed in Chapter 7.

Some Effective Coping Steps That You Can Take Right Now—or Whenever You Need Them

We all have far more coping resources available to us than we realize. The trouble is we don't know they're there. Whenever a crisis point in cancer seems altogether overwhelming, read through this list and discover the measures you can take. Coping isn't a single grand gesture; rather, it is a series of small steps that allow you to see clearly what needs to be done and to begin doing it. Here are some steps you can choose:

- *Lose the word* should. Any form of coping or dealing with illness is to be done to enhance the quality of one's life. Coping strategies are undertaken as *elective* opportunities, not guilt-driven expectations. Do them because they help you feel better, not because they fulfill an obligation.

- *Forget right or wrong.* There is no grading system to coping—no passing no failing, no graduating with honors. Coping is a process to be done by you, however you can.

- *Follow through on things.* If medication is prescribed, take it. Show up for therapy sessions. And keep your doctor's appointments—*every one of them.*

- *If you awaken in the morning feeling depressed, don't fight it.* Low moods are frequently their worst the first thing in the morning. Let yourself feel horrible. Cry, moan, feel as bad and sad as you wish. Then remind yourself that you will probably feel better as the day progresses. Use that realization to pull yourself out of bed, brush your teeth, make breakfast, and begin the tasks that give the day shape. This strategy lets the feelings out, but it keeps them from immobilizing you.

- *Take advantage of the times of the day and night when you feel best.* Depression and anxiety are commonly cyclic, peaking at certain times and declining at others. Use the times when you feel best to accomplish what you must.

- *Don't isolate yourself.* Some solitude is fine, but spending time with supportive family and friends helps keep low moods and anxiety at bay.

- *Stay away from people and situations that make you feel stressed.* If the neighbor two doors down makes you uncomfortable, stay away from her or him. Your life has sufficient stressors; don't add to them.

- *Divide big problems and tasks into small problems and tasks.* There is the old saying that an elephant is best eaten one bite at a time. If, instead of setting one huge goal—like achieving a complete remission of cancer—you break it into smaller, more easily achievable objectives—like showing up for next Wednesday's chemotherapy session—success is easier to achieve. And it is a positive feeling you can create and attain almost every day.

- *Demand less of yourself.* Don't be afraid to say no to added responsibilities. Give yourself permission to be sick. And forget perfectionism. Just getting something done is accomplishment enough.

- *If you are feeling low or anxious, put off major decisions.* The emotional reactions to cancer crises make it difficult to concentrate, and they skew your judgment skills. Delay major decisions about issues such as finances and your career until you feel calmer and more focused.

- *Listen to music and read.* Scientific studies show that music releases brain chemicals that contribute to a sense of well-being. Good poetry can have a similar effect. But you might want to choose more optimistic writers (e.g., Walt Whitman) over darker minds (e.g., Sylvia Plath). And don't be afraid of good escapist books like romance novels, sports biographies, and mysteries; indulge in them.

- *Avoid alcohol, as well as drugs not prescribed by your physician.* Alcoholics Anonymous has a saying: There is no problem so bad one drink won't make it worse. Alcohol and other drugs *seem* to offer escape, but in fact they can make you feel much worse, as if you are in a place from which there is no escape. This is particularly true if you are drinking while taking prescribed psychotropic medication, such as antianxiety drugs.

- *Connect with a support group for other people with cancer.* It's amazing how much better it can make you feel to realize you are not alone in your sleepless nights and fears of death and disability.

- *Eat ice cream.* We ought to respect our bodies through exercise and nutrition, but not to the deprivation of pleasure. The occasional ice-cream sundae or cheeseburger with lettuce, tomato, and a big slice of onion is good for our emotional souls.

- *Laugh!* Watch funny movies, read *Dilbert,* or go to the local comedy club. If it makes you laugh, do it. If you don't feel like laughing, try to summon up at least an occasional smile.

- *Spend time with children, animals, and plants.* Kids can be joyful and infectiously funny. Scientific studies have shown that the simple act of petting a dog or cat lowers blood pressure and heart rate. And gardening is a meditative activity that takes your mind off the problems you are facing and decreases the sensations of stress.
- *Keep a journal.* Making a daily diary entry gives you a way of recording how you are feeling and helps lend your emotions the shape of words. Often this simple act of emotional articulation can add to clarity and focus.
- *Buy flowers.* Place them so that you'll see them often. They'll remind you that, even with cancer, this is one beautiful world.
- *Pay attention to intimacy and love.* They are the most potent antidote to darkness in any of our lives. Friendships and family hold and heal our hearts.

PART TWO

❧

THE EMOTIONAL COURSE OF CANCER

3

ONE CRISIS ENDS,
ANOTHER BEGINS

CANCER REQUIRES YOU TO COPE, because a diagnosis of cancer causes a crisis in everyone who is diagnosed with it. Like losing a spouse, having a limb cut off in an accident, or watching a stock market crash wipe out your entire retirement nest egg, cancer imposes an obstacle to life goals that seems, at least for a time, too high and wide to be surmounted by your usual methods of solving problems. The result is confusion, disorganization, and a numbing inability to deal with the situation at hand in the tried-and-true ways that have worked in the past.

What makes cancer difficult is that it constitutes not one crisis but a series of crises. As you move through the course of the disease—from diagnosis to treatment to remission or recurrence—each change sets up the crisis anew. That is the bad news. The good news is that most people learn how to cope, both on their own and with a little help from their friends and the right professionals.

Is What I'm Feeling Normal?

The most common feelings coursing through patients dealing with cancer are anxiety and depression. Anxiety produces sweaty palms, a churning stomach, a racing heartbeat, and an intense sense of dread along with other psychological and physiological signs. Depression adds sadness to that. It causes bouts of crying, a low mood, lack of interest in such normally pleasurable pursuits as food and sex, and a lack of energy. Depression and anxiety often go hand in hand, so that the signs of one overlap with the other.

Cancer patients commonly ask their doctors whether their feelings of depression and anxiety are normal or whether they are the sign of some underlying psychological disorder that requires treatment. There are two parts to the answer. The first has to do with the difference between feelings and the symptoms of a disorder. The second has to do with understanding the emotional course of cancer, which we will look at in more detail as this chapter develops.

The distinction between feelings and symptoms can best be understood by an analogy with physical needs. Take thirst as an example. Everyone needs to drink a sufficient quantity of water each day. Engage in a hard game of tennis or a forty-mile bike ride on a warm day, and that need increases so greatly that it is easy to knock back a quart of cold water or sports drink in one giant gulp. But if that same thirst occurred without vigorous exercise and it was accompanied by blurry vision and poor wound healing, then it would be a potential symptom of diabetes.

The emotional crisis prompted by cancer induces a massive upwelling of emotions caused by the reality of the disease. Thoughts about disability and death are certain to lead to feelings of sadness. And if you are facing the prospect of surgery, chemotherapy, and/or radiation, it is only normal to feel anxiety over the pain, sickness, and difficult recovery these therapies entail. The low mood, sweaty palms, and lack of appetite that accompany thoughts about these realities are feelings on the order of a big thirst after a long exercise.

Feelings become symptoms of an underlying *disorder* only when they immobilize the individual, when they continue independently of thoughts about cancer, and when they are part of a constellation of other physical and psychological signs—in the same way that poor wound healing and blurry vision, when combined with an insatiable thirst, can signal diabetes. Returning to anxiety as an example, sweaty palms, a churning stomach, and a sense of impending doom at the thought of partial removal of the large intestine for treatment of colon cancer are hardly surprising. But finding oneself in the midst of an out-of-the-blue series of severe anxiety attacks that seem to have no link to current reality probably represents a symptom of panic disorder (which is discussed in detail in Chapter 7, as are other emotional disorders of cancer).

In understanding the feelings raised by cancer, it is important to realize that the disease throws you into a state of mourning. The life that you have known up to this point is passing away; a new stage of life is beginning. But your emotional mind is conservative; it wants to hang on to the life with which it is already acquainted. So when faced with the changes imposed by cancer, your psyche enters a state of grief, much as it would if a loved one had died. Cancer induces a natural and normal loss of what life has been and what life is expected to be. This emotional reaction is predictable, and, as with any process of grief, mourning, and bereavement, the psyche has to pass through the whole process in order to adapt, heal, and get on with living the new life.

So keep in mind that sadness and anxiety are not signs of weakness that could be surmounted if only you had sufficient strength of character to keep from giving in to your feelings. In fact, failure to express your feelings would be more likely to block your ability to gain access to the psychological resources you need to face the challenge of cancer and get on with your life.

I saw a striking example of this in a retired sixty-eight-year-old businessman named Mack who was diagnosed with colon cancer. Mack had been highly successful as an entrepreneur, and he had made himself into a wealthy man. However, Mack had long been a severe workaholic who ignored his personal life in favor of focusing on business. When a business deal went awry or when one of his adolescent sons began acting out, Mack withdrew emotionally, became both rigid and angry, and covered up his feelings with excessive eating, binge drinking, and cigar smoking. Bottling up his feelings, I suspected, lay behind his long medical history of chronic, severe headaches and indigestion (which only worsened his unrestrained forays into food, alcohol, and tobacco).

Mack followed the same maladaptive coping strategy when he was told that he had colon cancer. After going through the usual period of numbness that follows diagnosis, he withdrew emotionally, suppressed his feelings, acted passive and stoic with his surgeon and oncologist, and stayed up late at night to smoke cigars, drink snifter after snifter of brandy, and watch dark, depressing movies on the VCR. Mack never acknowledged his feelings, and he went through the cancer experience in a state of suspended emotion. There is no way to know whether Mack's response affected the course of his disease, but it certainly detracted from his quality of life and denied him the insights, understandings, and emotional development he might have achieved had he allowed himself to express the grief that was a natural reaction to the loss of his life as he had known it.

Because of the popular, and mistaken, notion that feelings of sadness and other low moods allow cancer to flourish and advance, many patients worry that their normal depressed feelings will affect treatment negatively. This is not the case, however. While it is true that an engaged, optimistic patient who takes cancer on with a fighting spirit generally feels better than someone who is stoic and passive, days when you feel dragged out and low-down are both normal and unavoidable. There is simply no evidence that temporary changes in mood influence odds for survival. In fact, sadness and anxiety are part of the healthy coping cycle and an inescapable aspect of facing up to a crisis and gathering the resources to surmount it. As mentioned earlier, it is far better to let the feelings emerge than it is to suppress them.

Understand, too, that there is no one "right" way to react emotionally to cancer. Given the wide range of personality styles in all of us, it is hardly surprising that different people react differently. Whereas some people respond with intense feelings, others in the same predicament find themselves more stoic, quiet, and reserved. This variation is normal and to be expected.

The Course That Cancer Takes

Cancer isn't a single crisis but a series of crises spaced out over time. The individual faces one challenge, adapts and copes, then finds himself or herself entering a new crisis. Understanding the normal emotional shape of each crisis will help you in coping with the range of feelings that arise at every step along the way. A thumbnail description of what happens during the course of the disease is presented here. Reactions and their time frames vary widely. As discussed in Chapter 7, there are many effective interventions to restore psychological equilibrium. In the chapters that follow, we will look more closely at each stage.

Diagnosis

Receiving a diagnosis of cancer plummets the individual into a period that has been termed *existential plight*. Fundamentally, he or she experiences a period of acute emotional distress that diminishes as he or she begins to accept the reality of the situation and begins to cope.

Typically this initial phase breaks into three phases. In the first, which usually lasts a week or so, the person experiences disbelief and denial, anxiety, and despair—perhaps focusing on one, perhaps alternating among all four. In denial or disbelief, the individual is convinced that the diagnosis is wrong and will soon be corrected or that the pathologist's report was based on the wrong slide. When despair takes over, the following thoughts predominate: "I just knew that spot of blood was cancer" or "It's stupid to get treated since I'm going to die anyway." Anxiety is characterized by obsessing and ruminating about the diagnosis and the fear it raises. Overall, the individual feels numb, almost as if he or she had left the body and were watching events from somewhere else. Sometimes people say things such as, "I had this feeling that all this was happening to somebody else."

The second phase, technically called dysphoria, commonly lasts several weeks but may go on longer. The numbness gives way to feelings that can be startlingly intense: sadness, irritability, depressed mood, lack of appetite, inability to sleep well or long enough, poor concentration, and difficulty in performing daily activities such as keeping up with a job or the housework. Above all else, one's usual ways of dealing with big problems are no longer working.

Then, in the third phase of coping or adaptation, some combination of old and new strategies begins to take effect. In most people, this begins about two to six weeks after diagnosis, although the range in time is quite variable. The individual adjusts to the new information, faces the issues, discovers reasons to feel optimistic, and resumes daily activities, whether getting on with the treatment plan or returning to family and occupational duties.

This cycle takes a different and more difficult turn in that rare person who learns that he or she has an extremely poor prognosis at the time of diagnosis. Some cancers present no symptoms until they are so far advanced that the usual therapies are ineffective. In this case, the individual has to come to terms not only with the disease but also with the potential of approaching death.

Treatment

Most cancers are treated with chemotherapy, surgery, radiation, immunotherapy, or a combination of these approaches. The beginning of each phase of treatment represents a new crisis. First, there is the seemingly endless wait before treatment begins; then there is the stressor of the treatment itself. Most patients enter treatment feeling relatively optimistic. They have a plan, they feel prepared to tolerate what they must put up with in order to survive, and they are looking for a cure.

Then comes the reality of the treatment. Surgical procedures can be painful and debilitating, and the side effects of chemotherapy and radiation are often noxious and upsetting. In addition, the individual has to face temporary or permanent changes in how the body looks and works. Hair may be lost, scars left, body parts removed. And the physical vulnerability and fatigue that accompany treatment can leave the individual feeling as if he or she has no resources left to fight with. Daily tasks are left undone, and roles in family and work that are central to self-worth may change in distressing ways. Typically, patients in treatment want time to move quickly; they would like to have this difficult part of their lives over and done with. Waiting, without an activity to provide a concentrated focus, can be immensely difficult and anxiety-provoking.

Still, treatment is hardly all bad. Some days are better than others, allowing moments of joy here and there, often in things that earlier would have been taken for granted—a phone call from an old friend, for example, or a really good novel.

Remission

After the rigors of treatment, remission of the cancer feels like a blessed relief, but it can also precipitate a new crisis. Residual effects of treatment may last months or even more than a year after the completion of chemotherapy or other interventions. Also, people feel as if they are now living in the predicament of Damocles, a figure from Greek antiquity who was forced to take part in a feast while sitting beneath a sword suspended from a single thread. Were that thread to break, Damocles would have been skewered alive. Surviving cancer can feel like that. You are alive and well, but this threat hangs over you, held aloft by the flimsiest of supports. No wonder that anxiety can well up like a spring tide. Many survivors find themselves frightened by the smallest change in their bodies ("Is that the cancer coming back?"), extremely fearful before follow-up visits to the oncologist, constantly seeking assurance that the cancer is indeed gone, and afraid that they are not being checked often enough or that they will lose contact with their physician who alone can save them. Simply seeing an article about cancer in a newspaper can precipitate an anxious reminder of the past and fear of the future.

From a positive perspective, often the crisis of remission centers on a new understanding of the meaning of an individual's life. In the crucible of diagnosis and treatment, many people discover the parts of their lives that don't work, only to be presented with the need to make a change when their lives are handed back to them. Julie was a prime example (see Chapter 2). Her remission presented a powerful dilemma: to go on living as she had been, hoping secretly for escape through death, or to create a new life based on the need to build her own core of personhood. Many patients find themselves in a less intense form of a similar dilemma. They have discovered significant realities about themselves, some of which hold the promise of changing the form and content of their lives. Now they have to consider whether they might change the way they have been living in order to adjust to these new insights.

Recurrence

The hard truth is that, in a percentage of cases, cancer does come back after an apparent remission. Research indicates that recurrence of cancer may be the most distressing event in the course of the disease. The shock, numbness, and waves of fear are similar to those at initial diagnosis, but this time there is a difference. Instead of focusing on a cure as the hoped-for end state, the individual must come to terms with the fact that the goal of treatment is control of the disease. Cancer has become not an illness to be cured but a chronic condition to be managed.

It is commonplace to feel vulnerable, frightened, frustrated, and betrayed. Many slip into the abyss of hopelessness and helplessness. Others grow angry at medical professionals. Many vacillate between a desire for immediate medical treatment, such as additional surgery or another cycle of chemotherapy or radiation, and despair that the treatment offers little utility over the long run and only adds discomfort, pain, and suffering. Typically, they are eventually able to focus their resources and commit themselves to finding the best course of action. At the same time, they must come to terms with the fact that the disease may not be controllable and that death could come sooner rather than later.

Advancing Disease

The next crisis comes when cancer responds poorly or not at all to treatment. Patients may seek out new treatment options, in the hope that there is a cure out there somewhere. Some sign up for clinical trials at university medical centers or seek alternative treatments that are grounded in scientific rigor. These are reasonable options, as they provide some realistic hope. However, others may become proponents of purported therapies that have yet to be shown to have any value in treating cancer, such as huge doses of vitamins, and sham medicines (for example, laetrile). The more desperately patients seek for the grail in the latest news report about a supposed miracle, the more likely they are to suffer significant distress marked by periods of anxiety and panic. The other option is for the patient to develop a new outlook on his or her condition, focusing more on care, physical comfort, and clear and open communication with loved ones. Realistic preparation for death, while itself a crisis, allows the individual to come to terms with his or her own life and achieve a kind of peace.

Running the Course of Cancer— Emotionally and Physically

The story of Mike, head football coach at a midsized college, illustrates fully how emotions change in the course of cancer, as one crisis is resolved, only to give way to another.

Mike was lucky in that he was both professionally and personally successful. Although he coached at an NCAA Division II school that gave no scholarships, he fielded a winning team year after year. He had no desire to move into the higher, more demanding realms of Division I football, preferring the hands-on coaching of a smaller, less demanding environment. Mike was a tough man who set high standards of fitness and accomplishment for his players, but he was also highly personable and dedicated to these young men, who flourished under his combination of discipline and warmth. On the family side of the ledger, he had done well too. After twenty-five years of marriage, he deeply loved his wife and was proud of his children—twin sons who had finished college and were beginning business careers and a daughter who was a senior in high school.

Mike was a fervent health advocate. He ate carefully and well, never smoked, drank moderately, kept his weight in line, and exercised passionately, cross-training in weight lifting, swimming, and cross-country bicycling. He assumed that he would get his usual clean bill of health when he went in for an annual physical at age fifty-three. Even when his physician said, "I think we need a closer look at your prostate," Mike tossed the remark off as nothing more than ordinary medical diligence. It surprised him when a blood test showed a markedly elevated level of the protein known as prostate-specific antigen (PSA), a possible indicator of cancer. But the real shock came after a biopsy of his prostate provided evidence of a cancerous tumor.

"I sat up at night and I thought there must have been a mistake. I had always been so religiously dedicated to my health that I felt like I was immortal. I knew I was supposed to die like everybody, but I assumed it would happen from a truck running me over when I was ninety-seven and still perfectly healthy. I never thought I'd be middle-aged, feeling fine, and told I had cancer."

As the numbness, shock, and denial wore off, anxiety and depression set in.

"I kept asking myself, 'Why me? What did I do wrong?' Then the really big question popped up: 'Am I going to die?' I'm supposed to be this tough guy, and the thought of death would pass through me, and I'd feel myself shaking like a leaf in a windstorm. Let me tell you, I was scared."

Mike was also confused, unable to focus, and withdrawn from his family and friends. When his urologist talked to him about treatment options, Mike was too mentally shaken to absorb the information and make any kind of choice. But as the first couple of weeks passed, he began to feel himself coming around.

"I realized this was just like a big football game. It's you against the other guy. Even when it hurts, you suck it up and keep going. I was determined to go after prostate cancer the same way."

Mike was lucky in that his tumor had been detected early—to all indications, before it had spread to any of the surrounding organs, so it could be treated with either radiation or surgery. In some cases, radical prostatectomy—complete surgical removal of the prostate, seminal vesicles, vas deferens, as well as local lymph nodes—can lead to difficulty holding urine, and it may also interfere with normal sexual function. Mike's urologist, however, told him that he was a candidate for a new nerve-sparing surgical technique that greatly lowers the risk of these complications. Radiation also carries some risk of complications, but it has a shorter recovery period, with no major incision to heal. After weighing the risks and benefits of radiation against the two surgical procedures, Mike decided on the radical prostatectomy.

"I wanted to be aggressive, to tackle the cancer as hard as I could," Mike said. "Surgery seemed to give me the best odds."

Still, contemplating the surgery, which entails a large incision in the abdomen and a lengthy hospital stay, caused Mike considerable anxiety. He had constant butterflies, could hardly eat or sleep during the three weeks leading up to his prostatectomy, and stumbled through his day-to-day duties, unable to focus on practices or game films.

"Then, for some reason, just before surgery I felt surprisingly calm," Mike explained. "I can remember feeling like that when I was playing football in college. The few days before a game, I was jumpy and edgy. But then, once I got on the field, I calmed down. The first quarter was about to begin. Surgery was much the same."

After surgery, Mike felt helpless, totally dependent on the nurses for everything. He hated the indignity of the catheter conducting urine out of his body as he healed, and he hated having to use a urinal in his bed for days after the catheter was removed. His feeling of dependency bothered him even more than the pain of recovery.

"I am a control-oriented person, the kind of guy who runs things. It's damn hard to feel like a baby who has to be taken care of by other people," Mike said. "And you can imagine my feelings about those stupid hospital gowns."

Once he was discharged, Mike was glad to get home. However, soon the reality of recovery from major surgery set in. For days, he was unable to walk, and even when he got back on his feet, he was too sore to exercise beyond a slow stroll down the block. He felt tired, uncomfortable, achy, too weakened to work or take any real part in the life of his family.

"I was out of the loop," he said. "My body and soul felt like they were stuck between gears and I was going no place."

Gradually, Mike's discomfort abated. He slowly regained his weight, appetite, and stamina and was able to move about, eventually returning to work and play. There was other good news too. His bladder control returned to normal, and his sexual capacity slowly increased as well.

Follow-up tests showed no cancer, and his PSA was zero, also indicating that there was no more prostate cancer in his body.

"My urologist was very pleased with himself," Mike said. "He said I was more likely to die from a heart attack during the two-minute drill in a championship game than from prostate cancer. He pronounced me cured."

For the most part, Mike himself felt cured. He returned to his work, family activities, and community involvement with new energy. Having felt supported by his wife and children, the football players, and the college during his illness, Mike felt as if he owed everyone a debt of gratitude. "My life had more meaning, more depth," he said. " I took nothing and no one for granted."

Yet there was an edge of fear, a knife of anxiety that twisted in Mike's soul from time to time.

"I noticed it first when I was listening to the TV news and anything about cancer came on. I'd feel really nervous, edgy. What bothered me most was a report about somebody famous dying of prostate cancer. I'd hear that news and I'd break out in a hot sweat all over. I'd think, 'Jeez, that could be me, and I wouldn't even get on the news.'"

That same anxiety heightened whenever Mike had a checkup with his physician. "One time, my doc screwed up his face and I thought, 'Oh no, it's back.' Then he looked at me and said, 'Your athlete's foot is flaring up. Start using a fungicide every morning.' I realized I was just scared of that damn cancer coming back."

It has been three years since Mike's initial diagnosis, and he remains cancer-free.

"It's funny now. Not a day goes by that I don't think of prostate cancer, sometimes with fear, sometimes with sadness, sometimes even with relief. But the truth of the matter is that I've come to a point where it doesn't scare me much. The disease just doesn't interfere with my life anymore. I'm focused more on getting on with the things that matter, like football and my family, than I am worrying about this disease. I'm ready to take what comes."

Mike's story illustrates extremely healthy coping and adjusting to cancer. It is important to note, though, that he didn't adjust once and for all to the disease and move on. Rather, he progressed from crisis to crisis, managing a new set of emotions at each turn. Now we will look at each step in that emotional process, beginning with diagnosis.

4

COPING WITH THE DIAGNOSIS

YEARS AGO, A MAJOR INSURANCE COMPANY ran a magazine advertising campaign featuring wonderfully whimsical cartoon drawings of people a split second away from total disaster. One of them showed a well-dressed man strolling along a city street as a grand piano was plummeting toward him. The humor in the ad came from the way it suspended disaster: The piano seemed to hang in air, while the man only a few feet below had no idea of the fate he was about to meet. It was funny.

But when the piano hits, it's no longer funny—which is exactly what happens when you or a loved one receives a diagnosis of cancer. Suddenly, out of the blue, the falling piano has crashed down. You are trapped under its full weight: surprised, hurting everywhere, uncertain what has happened, knowing full well that the life you have been living has just changed in a way you can't even begin to understand.

The Emotional Impact

Most people go through three distinct stages as the impact of a cancer diagnosis sinks in and the emotional consequences make themselves known.

Stage 1: Denial, Depersonalization, and Dread

Even when Roberta, a forty-three-year-old married mother of two school-age children and a personal injury attorney, was told that the small mass in her right breast needed to be removed for microscopic examination, she didn't get excited. She knew the odds were in her favor: Five out of six breast lumps aren't cancerous.

A routine mammogram revealed a suspicious shadow, which Roberta's gynecologist checked with a procedure called fine-needle aspiration. The breast often contains cysts, which are sac-like structures that fill with liquid and are seldom cancerous. If a thin needle inserted into a breast lump taps into fluid and the cells are nonmalignant, then the lump is rarely cancer. But Roberta's physician said that her aspiration was inconclusive, and he advised that the lump be removed by a surgeon and extensively examined in a pathology lab. The procedure, done with mild sedation and a local anesthetic, was no more uncomfortable than having a tooth extracted—except, Roberta said, "I wasn't real keen on somebody handling sharp instruments anywhere near my chest. Still, I decided to grin and bear it. Turns out it wasn't that bad."

With her husband, she came back three days later for the lab report. After the usual how-are-you's, the gynecologist settled into his chair, looked at Roberta earnestly across his desk, and said, "The bad news is it's cancer."

"I never heard the good news," she said. "The minute the word *cancer* was spoken, I blanked out. Whatever my doctor said, it just floated in air like these balloons I couldn't catch or comprehend. Then, when I began to make out what he was saying, I was certain he wasn't talking about me. No, he was talking about somebody else—I just knew it! I remember he began listing all these treatment options and mentioning the names of surgeons and oncologists, and I wanted to say, 'You've got the wrong person. This is silly. I don't need a surgeon—and certainly not an oncologist!'" This response is a classic and typical example of *denial*—that is, disavowing a reality that is too painful to accept.

Roberta was also experiencing something psychiatrists call *depersonal-*

ization: a feeling that one has moved outside one's own body. Depersonalization is a common response to such trauma as being trapped in battle, caught in the midst of a terrible car accident, or subjected to rape or torture. Because the mind cannot grasp such an overwhelming experience, it extracts itself from reality as a method of self-defense.

With Roberta, as with most people who depersonalize, the feeling of being outside herself lasted only a short time. Even by later that night, the reality of cancer in her life was beginning to sink in. Reality brought with it anxiety.

"I had this general feeling of *dread*. At times, I felt like I was floating on an ocean of fear, floating wherever its cruel currents took me," Roberta said. "My hands would suddenly start to tremble, for no apparent reason at all. Anytime I tried to concentrate, my mind jumped immediately to thoughts of cancer, dying, and death. Those first few nights were absolutely the worst. I thought for sure I'd never sleep again. Every night, the fears and dreads just got worse. I'm a very independent person, but I kept waking my husband up to hold me, just to tell me things were still all right."

What Roberta experienced typifies the first stage in the crisis of a cancer diagnosis. Emotionally knocked over by the diagnosis, the individual responds with denial and depersonalization, which then transforms into an anxiety characterized by obsession and rumination. In Roberta's case, this initial response lasted about a week, which is fairly typical. Sometimes it lasts longer, and sometimes it ends sooner, depending on the individual's psychological makeup and the type and severity of the cancer.

Stage 2: Depression and Dismal Thoughts

At the next stage of her emotional response to the diagnosis, Roberta slipped into sadness.

"I had crying spells and nervousness—not something I normally experience. Above all else, I felt helpless and hopeless. And nothing interested me. I love good food and wine, and my husband was sweet enough to cook some of my favorite dishes, but after a bite or two I was done. My husband and I really enjoy each other's bodies, yet the very idea of sex was unthinkable. I just didn't care. I obsessed endlessly about death, about cancer taking away my life. I hadn't told the kids what was going on, but they sensed the tension in the air, and the kids tried to cheer me up the way kids do. I smiled at them with no enthusiasm, then broke out crying. I was trying to hide it, but they knew something was very wrong."

Roberta still had trouble sleeping, and her concentration was almost nonexistent. She tried to continue her job at the law firm, then discovered that she simply didn't have the intellectual stamina to work on the cases assigned to her. Wisely, she took a brief sick leave until she settled down emotionally.

In this second part of the emotional response to diagnosis, the reality of cancer is becoming part of the individual's emotional self-image. Since our culture closely links cancer to death's darkest forces, thoughts focus on the possible end of life. Some people find this doubly disturbing, assuming— falsely—that thinking about death is a prediction that they will indeed imminently die.

Stage 3: Return to "Normalcy"

About five weeks after the diagnosis, Roberta began to find the strength to cope. Her appetite improved, and she could sleep, first for a few hours, then all night long. Her concentration was good enough that she could help her kids with homework again. For the first time since her diagnosis, her sexuality reawakened, and she and her husband picked up erotically where they had left off. Roberta found herself better able to consider her treatment options and integrate them into her own needs and personality.

"Sometimes I still felt nervous and I would 'overthink.' It's something attorneys do; we look at a situation from every possible angle, so we won't be outflanked in court. I was doing that. Still, it worked for me; that's my style. I really studied the options. When I selected a lumpectomy with follow-up chemotherapy, I felt as confident as I could that I was choosing the approach that gave me the best odds against the disease with the fewest side effects."

Essentially, Roberta had returned to the psychological baseline where she had begun. Indeed, this is the arc that most people trace when first confronted by cancer. They move through the denial and dread of the first stage, then enter the pronounced sadness and negative thinking of the second, and then return finally to an emotional place not altogether different from where they began. In this third stage, the individual adjusts and copes, faces the issues presented by the disease, begins to feel better, and returns to such central activities as family and professional life. And although most people return close to their emotional baseline, as we shall see throughout the book, brief periods of anxiety and depression are often a part of living with cancer. Fortunately, if this is known, coping may be easier and new ways of adapting may be learned. The amount of time each step takes depends on a number of factors that vary from person to person.

Factors That Affect How You Adjust to the Diagnosis

Everyone who receives a cancer diagnosis reacts to it in his or her own unique way. A number of personal and psychological factors play into the differences that lead one individual to react differently from another.

Emotional Differences

No challenge places the fear of death, of losing existence, in front of us more than a diagnosis of cancer. Since this fear cuts deeply into the roots of the individual's psychology, the way that individual reacts has a great deal to do with his or her belief system and psychological history.

RELIGIOUS AND ETHICAL BELIEFS

The widowed mother of four and the grandmother of twelve, Kate was eighty years old when she learned that her chronic bouts of indigestion were due to an aggressive colon cancer. At first, she was overwhelmed with the knowledge of her own mortality. Like Roberta, she first felt disbelief and dread. Then she moved through the predictable insomnia and depression into the third phase of acceptance and adjustment with unusual speed. The reason, she explained to me, was her religion.

Raised an Irish Catholic, Kate had always been devout. She said the rosary daily, attended mass on weekdays as well as Sundays, and observed Lent with great care. Catholicism had given her long life the structure and meaning of repeated ritual. It also gave her a framework into which to place her own current situation. Life, she knew, entailed suffering. The key to the Gospel was that Jesus was born to die on the cross and only then to rise from the dead. Cancer was like the cross to her; it was the suffering she had to pass through to enter the better life she believed lay beyond. Above all else, cancer was beyond her control. It was God's will.

"Having cancer allows me to practice my faith," said Kate.

And she wasn't bitter. "I've lived long, and I've both loved and been loved. I have wonderful children and grandchildren. I feel sad sometimes, but I don't have anything to regret."

Orthodox belief is not the only antidote to the fear of death that cancer raises. Any belief system, even a secular one, that provides support and meaning can be of great value.

Jessica was another patient in her eighties, also widowed, also diagnosed with an aggressive cancer—in her case, in the pancreas. She was less emotional than Kate, more a creature of the intellect than the heart. Trained originally as a physician, Jessica had retired from medicine in her fifties and devoted herself to painting. Raised as a mainline Protestant, she abandoned religion during college and took up agnosticism when she found herself drawn to existentialism. At first, she entered the dark and unforgiving vision of Jean-Paul Sartre, then moved into the more humane worldview of Albert Camus. The writers who gave her the greatest solace were the psychiatrists Rollo May and Victor Frankl. Both embraced free will and choice as the key demands of human life, and stressed the need for each of us to find meaning in our daily lives. Jessica particularly respected Frankl. A European Jew who survived the Holocaust as a concentration camp inmate, he refused to give up the search for meaning under even the most dire circumstances.

"If Frankl could deal with the Nazis," Jessica said, "I figured I could deal with cancer."

Having been a physician as well as a student of philosophy and an artist, Jessica recognized the inevitability of death. "There's no reason to moan about what has to be," she said. "Not that I see any reason to go before I need to or to be uncomfortable in the meantime. Still, dying is part of the big picture. Nobody gets away without doing it."

Able to understand her emotional needs and buoyed by a belief system that made her at once accepting of the inevitable and personally responsible for her sense of meaning, Jessica was able to adapt to her disease, choose among the treatments offered, and select the therapy that fit best with who she was.

FEELINGS ABOUT DEATH

Religion alone may not be enough to overcome a particularly traumatic encounter with death, especially in early life.

Deborah was only eight when she watched her thirty-year-old mother die of a brain aneurysm. One moment her mother was preparing dinner, the next she had collapsed on the floor. Deborah remembered that day as the worst in her life. Raised as a Conservative Jew, she recalled the procession to the cemetery with its lines of headstones inscribed in Hebrew and the dark-clad mourners filling the house to observe the ritual mourning period, or shiva, that followed.

Deborah's father never fully recovered from his wife's unexpected death. Bereft and depressed, he remained alone and isolated for the rest of his life. He lived to be an old man, but the cloud of darkness never lifted from him. Although Deborah maintained that she loved her father, she could not consciously admit to herself that she felt as if he also had abandoned her, just as her mother had.

Deborah developed a deeply morbid fear, or phobia, of death and the loss it entails. To defend herself against the consuming feelings that even the faintest thought of death raised, Deborah threw herself into her studies with rigid expectations and a tendency to overthink all her tasks, and later into her professional career as an academic historian. Still the death phobia sometimes raised its ugly head. When a university colleague or a member of her extended family died, Deborah was too consumed by fear to even think about attending the funeral.

From the moment Deborah was diagnosed with cancer, anxiety paralyzed her. Her fears of death took many forms, filling her days with endless ruminations on the coldness of nonbeing and her nights with nightmares full of monsters and dark caverns. Although not a devoutly religious person, Deborah had remained connected to the Jewish community and attended synagogue regularly. This connection to tradition and ritual gave her little comfort, though; Deborah's death phobia was simply too powerful.

After about a month, Deborah's thinking underwent an unusual change. Inexplicably, numbers and colors filled her mind and dominated her mental activity. An intellectual by style and an academic by profession, Deborah knew these obsessions were abnormal or irrational thoughts, but she could not control them. She repeated the names of the primary colors over and over. Then she counted numbers, sometimes odd, sometimes even, for hours on end. She checked the locks in her house again and again, sometimes six or eight times in an hour, even when she knew no one had entered or left by any of the doors since the last check. When she was driving, she could not keep herself from constantly thinking she had just run over a child without realizing it. Then she'd backtrack along her route to look for a small, crushed body in the street. Finding nothing didn't reassure her. Next time she went out in her car, she did the same thing.

The anxiety building around these irrational thoughts and behaviors led Deborah to believe that she was going crazy. Finally, the fear of her potential insanity so overwhelmed her one night that she phoned a hospital hot line. After listening to Deborah's list of repetitive thoughts and actions, a caring social worker on the other end of the line told her that she probably had a treatable mental disease known as obsessive-compulsive disorder.

Referred to me for therapy, Deborah learned that even though her obsessions (such as the preoccupation with numbers and primary colors) and her compulsions (such as checking the house locks repeatedly and doubling back over her driving route to find dead children) were uncomfortable, they served a purpose: Her symptoms were a desperate, unconscious attempt to gain control over her fears of death, which stemmed from a lifelong phobia. When Deborah was thinking about numbers, at least she wasn't thinking about dying.

PERSONALITY TYPES AND DISORDERS

Deborah had nursed a death phobia and an obsessive-style personality for decades. Most of the time, she handled it well; directing her energy into her demanding academic work kept her too busy to break out into a hot sweat at the thought of the end of life. But cancer stripped away her ordinary defense mechanisms and bared the old fear to the point where it bloomed into an emotional disorder (which will be discussed in Chapter 7).

Cancer does this again and again, on a scale ranging from the minor to the major. At the extreme end of the scale, a cancer diagnosis often drives the individual into the most maladaptive aspects of his or her personality. As we noted in the discussion of basic personality types in Chapter 2, each personality type in its most florid expression becomes a psychiatric disorder. The obsessive-compulsive disorder, for example, is a rigidly consuming version of the personality type that is punctual, orderly, and highly responsible. Typically, the high stress brought on by a cancer diagnosis causes people to become, in a sense, even more of what they usually are.

This is the case even with people who have worked hard to overcome the maladaptive aspects of their personalities. For example, I have seen individuals with dependent personalities who have become strikingly independent and self-assured and confident. Then, when a cancer diagnosis is delivered, all that hard-won independence and self-direction is lost. The individual moves toward his or her original personality type—a change psychiatrists call regression. Suddenly, the once-independent person fears being alone, cries when a family member leaves the house, and cannot make up his or her mind on even the simplest of decisions. In most cases, however, this regression is short-lived. As the individual moves through the stages of the emotional reaction to the diagnosis and begins to integrate this reality into his or her psychological worldview, he or she is again able to cope. The dependent person, for example, stops fearing solitude, tolerates the family's coming and goings, and ultimately makes an informed choice about treatment options.

A cancer diagnosis is also a way of bringing previously treated disorders to the fore. People who have suffered major depression and succeeded in treatment, for example, are more likely to slip back into the disorder when they receive a cancer diagnosis than individuals who have no history of depression. The root of Deborah's obsessive-compulsive disorder behavior was the phobic fear of death that had long plagued her. Exacerbated by the cancer diagnosis, her phobia flowered into a complex disorder.

The Waiting Game

One of the most emotionally demanding aspects of a cancer diagnosis is waiting. It often begins with a period of uncertainty occasioned by a physician's suspicion, an abnormal test result, or an unexplainable symptom. Follow-up tests, including biopsies, ultrasounds, or exploratory surgeries, are often required to make the diagnosis. The patient has to wait for the tests to be performed, then wait again for the results. Then even when the cancer diagnosis is clear, more tests may be needed in order to determine if the cancer has spread, since the extent of the disease often determines treatment options. That means even more waiting. And once a treatment choice has been made, there's yet another wait until treatment actually begins.

Nobody likes waiting. I've yet to meet anyone who actually enjoys standing in the checkout line at the grocery store, sitting in traffic, or lying in a dentist's chair in anticipation of a root canal. Cancer patients have to put up with more than their fair share of waiting. For some personality types, this aspect of the disease is particularly galling.

An apt example of this was Rob, a stockbroker and married father of three who was forty years old when I first saw him. It was obvious from the moment I spotted him in my waiting room that he was restless. Sitting in a chair, he shuffled his legs constantly, cracked his knuckles, and ran his fingers through his hair. The muscles in his face were drawn and tight, and his eyes darted about the room.

From Rob's oncologist I knew that he had a carcinoma of the thyroid gland, a highly treatable type of cancer. Complaining of hoarseness that had lasted about a year, Rob went to his family doctor, who found a suspicious nodule on the thyroid gland, which is located near the base of the throat and produces a number of important hormones. The inevitable tests followed: blood work, a thyroid scan, and a biopsy of the gland. Although the diagnosis was cancer, the good news was that this form of the disease responds extremely well to treatment and spreads very slowly. Rob was scheduled to have thyroid surgery in about two weeks, and he would then be given radiation as a follow-up treatment. Following surgery, he would need to take thyroid medication to replace the lost hormones. Except for that inconvenience, it was highly likely that Rob would have a normal life span free of any return of the cancer.

Yet it was clear from his demeanor that Rob was highly agitated. When I asked him how I could help, he came right to the point. "It's this waiting, the endless waiting," he said, the words bursting from him. "It's two more weeks till the surgery, and then I'll have to wait around to recover enough from that for the radiation to begin. I honestly can't stand it."

I agreed with him that waiting isn't easy, not for anyone.

"For me, it's worse," he said, anticipating my next question before I could even ask it. "I'm a take-charge, go-to kind of guy. That's why I'm a success as a stockbroker. I love the action, making decisions on the spot, the scorecard I get at the end of each day when I can see how much money I made or lost. For me the market can't move fast enough."

"What do you do in your spare time?" I asked.

"Competitive bicycle racing. In a former life I probably did the Tour de France."

Rob's personality didn't fit well with the slow-moving, bureaucratic reality of our medical system. In fact, when I asked him to describe what his experience had been like, he talked much more about waiting around for the tests, postponed appointments with surgeons and oncologists, and the delay before surgery than about the cancer itself. Like everyone who receives a cancer diagnosis, Rob had gone through the expected depersonalization, denial, and despair. Then, when he fully realized how treatable his disease was, his anxiety about the cancer itself largely dissipated. He wasn't looking forward to the removal of his thyroid, but he was more anxious about waiting out those two weeks than about the pain, fatigue, and weakness he was certain to experience during recovery.

As Rob and I worked together to untangle the source of his anxiety, it became more and more clear that the cause of his emotional reaction lay in his approach to the world. Because he was a take-charge, action-oriented man, Rob detested uncertainty, passivity, and the inability to control his own destiny. Cancer was serving him major portions of all three. The more often and the longer he waited, be it for a lab test, a doctor's appointment, or surgery, the more out of control Rob felt. Cancer made him passive rather than active, dependent on others instead of independent—a complete reversal of his usual way of being. Rob tried to deny the depth of his feelings, but they had broken past his denial to swell into a powerful anxiety.

Over the course of several psychotherapy sessions, Rob's anxiety level lessened. Not that he came to enjoy waiting; nobody does. Rather, Rob gave himself permission to be passive and not in control, to be sad, and to express his feelings. In his own way, he came to terms with the emotional reality of his disease.

The Stress of Second Opinions and Treatment Options

Another difficult aspect of the cancer diagnosis is the need to gather as much information as possible about the disease and decide how to go about treating it. People often find themselves facing difficult and demanding choices at a time when they feel emotionally unable to make decisions.

A fifty-year-old businessman and former Eagle Scout, Stu was surprised to find that the swollen glands in his neck and his excessive fatigue were due to a cancer of the lymph system known as non-Hodgkin's lymphoma.

He was such a straight arrow in all his lifestyle choices that he considered himself immune from such problems as cancer and heart disease. Once he let the reality of his diagnosis sink in, he found himself overwhelmed by the choices he had to make. As Stu's oncologist laid out his medical situation, he learned there were at least four available treatments, each with its pros and cons.

The first was a standard, well-tested chemotherapy protocol known as CHOP (cyclophosphamide, doxorubicin, vincristine, prednisone), a treatment using four drugs whose effectiveness against non-Hodgkin's lymphoma has been well proven in scientific studies. The second choice was chemotherapy plus the immunotherapy drug Rituxan, which activates the patient's own immune system to target cancer cells. Immunotherapy is very promising, but since it is still relatively new, its long-term effects are less well known than those of chemotherapy, and there are also side effects. The third option, combined chemotherapy and radiation, uses the rays emitted by radioactive material to kill fast-dividing cancer cells, which are particularly vulnerable to radiation. Finally, a bone marrow transplant was the most aggressive treatment option, which is actually a mechanism to permit massive chemotherapy, radiation, or both. Bone marrow is removed from the patient and cleansed of all cancer cells. Then the patient is subjected to potent rounds of chemotherapy and or radiation to kill any remaining cancer cells in the body. The cleansed bone marrow is then reintroduced into the patient. Bone marrow transplant — and a newer, similar procedure called stem cell transplant —can be dramatically successful. They are also arduous, time-consuming, and uncomfortable because of their side effects and a long recovery period. Occasionally they can prove fatal—and they don't always work.

In Stu's case, he left the oncologist's office weighed down with brochures on each treatment option. His oncologist, a bright, Ivy League–trained doctor, admitted that she was conservative and favored standard chemotherapy. Still, she suggested that Stu visit some other experts and get their opinions. She even gave him their phone numbers. And thus the parade of second opinions began.

Stu went to a major cancer center, where an imperious, self-assured, and totally arrogant research scientist informed him that immunotherapy was the only real option. The scientist also invited Stu to take part in a research study. There was a catch, however. Since this was a controlled double-blind study—in which neither doctors nor patients knew exactly which drugs they were giving or receiving—Stu had a 50 percent chance of getting immunotherapy and a 50 percent chance of receiving standard chemotherapy. Confused and frightened, Stu said no.

"I didn't like this guy's know-it-all style," Stu said. "And I wanted to make a choice, not be a guinea pig in somebody else's experiment."

Next he visited a lymphoma expert at a teaching hospital in another major city. This physician outlined the same four basic choices that his own oncologist had, and admitted that no one really knew which one was best.

"Not comforting," Stu said. "So I kept looking. I wanted certainty."

He didn't find any. Even though each of the next three physicians he spoke with had their own beliefs in what worked best, they admitted that the data really weren't in yet.

"This is nothing like strep throat," Stu said. "The doctor writes a prescription, says, 'Take this,' you do it, and the strep throat goes away in three days. My kind of cancer is altogether different. There's no sure thing."

Wrapped in uncertainty and anxiety, Stu felt paralyzed. He simply couldn't make up his mind. So he talked to his oncologist about a psychiatric consultation, and he came to see me.

Working together, he and I revisited the stunning experience of the diagnosis and then faced the array of unclear choices about treatment. As I got to know him better, one thing about Stu stood out: He took responsibility.

"You've always been an Eagle Scout," I said to him. "The kind of man who's resourceful, hardworking, never shirks his duty. You're a stand-up fellow. But this responsibility isn't all yours. It's more of a shared governance with your physician. Doctors don't have exact answers, but we do have hopeful options."

In a fairly short time, Stu came to understand that there was no right or wrong decision. Rather, there were alternatives, each with advantages and disadvantages.

Keeping this in mind, Stu went back to his first oncologist to review the options. They decided—together—to try immunotherapy, combined with standard chemotherapy. In part, this choice fit with Stu's personal style: He was willing to take risks but liked having the tried-and-true as part of the solution. Stu could now let his anxiety go and gather his psychological resources to deal with treatment.

In a cancer diagnosis, second opinions are more the rule than the exception. Requesting additional input is good in that it gives the patient a feeling of control, but this search can also precipitate massive stress and discomfort. Some people seek second opinions endlessly and obsess too long over their choices, often postponing treatment. Conversely, others may be too shy or dependent to ask for outside help, possibly subjecting themselves to a treatment regimen without knowing the available alternatives. The best path lies somewhere in between. The more complex your treatment options and the more your personality requires information, the more opinions you should seek. Once you understand the choices, it's time to decide, selecting an alternative that fits best with your personality style.

Survival Rates

A note on statistics and survival rates: At some point after you receive a diagnosis, you will discuss with your doctor (or read about) your chances of remission or cure. These are discussed in terms of survival rates, or, how many people with a certain type of cancer are living after 5 years, 10 years, and so forth. Remember, these are simply averages and each individual is unique. Keep in mind, survival rates are often outdated. They may not include the newest treatments or the most up-to-date options. Be careful not to embrace such statistics without a grain of salt and a pound of hope!

Guidelines for Coping Better After Your Diagnosis

These approaches and reminders can make it much easier to get through the initial stages of cancer:

- *Get administrative and secretarial help from your friends.* The emotions surrounding diagnosis can be so powerful that you are likely to miss important information. Take a friend, spouse, partner, or other family member along to serve as an extra pair of ears and take notes. If you receive a diagnosis or other information over the phone, have your helper listen in. Alternatively, use a tape recorder whenever you see a physician to talk about test results and treatment options.

- *Don't be afraid to ask.* If you are unclear about something, call the physician back and get it straightened out. Save yourself from worrying over a misunderstanding.

- *Let yourself feel your feelings and speak them out loud to your loved ones.* This applies to whatever your feelings are—fear, sadness, anger, hostility, anxiety, and even hope. Allow the feeling to express itself, and let those close to you know how you feel.

- *Balance solitude with connection.* The sadness that follows a cancer diagnosis often drives people into being alone. Some time by yourself is fine, but don't overdo it. Being with people you are close to can help mitigate unhappy feelings and remind you of your place in the world.

- *If you can't sleep and you're overwhelmed by anxiety, get help.* Short-term use of a sleeping aid or antianxiety medication prescribed by your doctor won't result in addiction. One important caveat: Use medication to *alleviate* symptoms, such as sleeplessness, not to take feelings away.

- *Recognize that you have not been found "guilty."* You *didn't* cause your cancer. The disease *isn't* your fault. Even in cases where those is a link between heavy smoking and lung cancer, excessive guilt has no emotional value and only diminishes self-respect. Let it go!

- *Avoid excessive alcohol.* If you enjoy a glass of wine with dinner, by all means let yourself have it. But don't go on a binge. Alcohol may seem to provide short-term relief, but in fact it only makes emotional dilemmas worse. If you're on medication, check with your physician or pharmacist about possible interactions with alcohol.

- *Let your loved ones nurture you.* They're doing you a favor, and you're doing them one. Cancer profoundly affects the people close to you. Letting them help you gives them the opportunity to take some measure of control over the situation.
- *Realize that thinking about death is normal and natural.* It doesn't mean that you will die. Rather, you are facing the fear of death implicit in a cancer diagnosis.
- *Tell yourself several times a day that this is a crisis; it will pass.* This reassurance is only intellectual, but the point is true. As you move through the crisis of a diagnosis, your feelings will change. Reminding yourself of the crisis nature of your situation will lay the groundwork for returning to normal.
- *If difficult feelings persist and you don't seem to be moving on, ask for professional help.* Psychotherapy, medication, and support groups can be important aspects of your fight against cancer.
- *Rely on your coping skills.* Use the various techniques detailed in Chapter 2. Then keep using the ones that work for you.

Knowing When to Ask for Psychiatric Help

As we discussed in Chapter 3, feelings are one thing, but symptoms of an emotional disorder are quite another. From the inside looking out, however, the distinction can be a hard one to make. These guidelines can help you decide if and when your feelings have crossed over into symptoms of a disorder and professional help is advised:

- *Extreme indecision about treatment.* As we saw in Stu's case, once you have the basic facts and alternative treatments in hand, it's time to make a decision. If you find you simply can't but instead obsess for weeks about the choice, it's likely that your fears are getting in the way.
- *Sustained or extreme conflict with family, friends, or physicians.* Fights with the people around you and those involved in your treatment can signal an underlying emotional conflict that needs to be dealt with.

- *History of an emotional disorder, especially depression or anxiety.* Even if you have been managing your disorder well, a cancer diagnosis is often likely to push you into a recurrence. It's wise to consult with the professional who has treated you, even before any problems arise.
- *Sexual disorders.* If you have been sexually active before diagnosis, it is likely that in the immediate emotional crisis of diagnosis you will lose interest in sex. Usually, however, erotic desire comes back as you work through the crisis and you return to your psychological baseline. A complete lack of interest over a period of weeks or months can indicate that the crisis is continuing and you need professional help.
- *Suicidal thoughts.* The desire to end one's life is not a normal response to cancer. An excellent study by a team of Canadian researchers headed by Harvey Chochinov, M.D., found that the desire for death, even among terminally ill patients, is a sign of severe depression, which is very treatable and is not an inevitable result of the disease.
- *Symptoms of anxiety or depression.* The two most common mental disorders during diagnosis are adjustment disorder and major depression. They are complex enough that we will look at each here, and in detail in Chapter 7:

  - Adjustment Disorder
    Adjustment disorder refers to a body of significant emotional symptoms that develop in response to an identifiable stressor, of which a diagnosis of cancer diagnosis is a prime example. The symptoms arise within three months of the stressful event, and they exceed what would be considered normal for that type of stress. Thus, sleeplessness for a week following a diagnosis of cancer is clearly normal; sleeplessness for two months isn't. The symptoms are so pronounced that they interfere with the individual's ability to carry on his or her professional or occupational duties and family life. Adjustment disorder can include symptoms of anxiety (primarily a state of overwrought mood), symptoms of depression (principally a state of extreme sadness), or both.

- Major Depression

Everyone—and particularly someone who has just received a diagnosis of cancer—goes through low moods. That's normal; major depression isn't. In this disorder, the low mood is extreme in both expression and duration, and it represents a change from the person's normal behavior. Symptoms are so pronounced that they make it very difficult for the individual to hold a job or participate in family life.

Depression is likely in cases where an individual has experienced at least five of the following symptoms—including depressed mood (1) or loss of interest in routine activities (2)—nearly every day for at least two weeks:

1. Depressed mood, typically indicated by bouts of crying and feelings of emptiness and sadness

2. Diminished pleasure in daily activities that previously gave pleasure, such as eating, professional work, lovemaking, reading, listening to music, playing games, taking the dog for a walk, and so forth

3. Significant weight loss without dieting, or a sudden increase or decrease in weight

4. Sleeping too much, too little, or sporadically

5. A marked speeding up or slowing down of body activity, expressed as constant agitation or by sitting around the house all day and doing nothing

6. Fatigue or lack of energy

7. Feelings of worthlessness or guilt that are excessive and inappropriate ("I caused this cancer. It's all my fault.")

8. Diminished ability to think or concentrate; indecisiveness

9. Repeated thoughts of death, or planning or attempting suicide

How to Find Help

Some people with cancer experience the expected normal emotional symptoms that accompany diagnosis and nothing more. For them, family and friends provide sufficient support. Still, a significant number of people with cancer find that support from family and friends falls short, and they want or need professional help in dealing with the emotions that arise as they attempt to come to grips with their diagnosis. If you are one of these people, keep two things in mind: (1) *selecting the right kind of professional* and (2) *finding the right individual to work with.*

Helping Professionals

A number of different types of licensed professionals deal with emotional and mental disorders. Each profession has particular training requirements and specific strengths.

Psychiatrists are medical doctors who have graduated from an accredited four-year medical school and have completed at least four years of psychiatric residency. They have studied the physiology and anatomy of the human body and have taken clinical rotations while in medical school in areas ranging from surgery to pediatrics to obstetrics. During residency they train in a wide range of treatments including psychotherapy and pharmacotherapy (use of medications). Since they are physicians, psychiatrists can order lab tests and prescribe medications.

Psychologists aren't medical doctors. Rather, they earn a doctorate in a university or professional school graduate program, which takes from three to seven years to complete. Some psychologists hold a Sci.D. degree, which indicates a clinical orientation in their training. Others have a Ph.D., which may point to more of a research focus. Following the doctorate, a psychologist has to complete an internship in a hospital or organized health care setting and at least one year of supervised clinical work. Since they are not physicians, psychologists are not licensed to prescribe medication or order lab tests. Psychologists primarily use various forms of psychotherapy—also known as talk therapy—in their work.

Licensed clinical social workers (L.C.S.W.s) also use psychotherapy. They have either a master's degree (M.S.W.) or a doctorate (D.S.W.) in social work with a focus on psychotherapy, and they have undergone an internship and supervised clinical experience that usually lasts three years.

A number of states license *therapists* who have graduated from master's programs with an emphasis on psychotherapy and psychology and completed a clinical internship. In California, for example, these professionals are known as marriage and family therapists (M.F.T.s). Other states license registered nurses (R.N.s) who have completed additional training in psychotherapy. In all states, members of the clergy can engage in pastoral counseling, also known as spiritual direction.

All other things being equal, the key professional in treating the mental disorders surrounding cancer should be a psychiatrist. Because they are medical doctors, psychiatrists are well equipped to understand the impact of disease on the body and the psyche, and the effects of medication. Psychologists, L.C.S.W.s, and similarly trained therapists also can be very useful when psychotherapy is needed. They pay close attention to the emotional issues in mental disorders.

Finding a Psychiatrist

Actually, it's easier to find a good psychiatrist than you might think. But rather than simply using the phone book—which tells you nothing about credentials or experience—ask around. Here are the people to consult:

- *Your oncologist.* Since the oncologist deals with cancer patients daily, he or she may well recognize when a psychiatric consultation is indicated and may provide a recommendation. Discuss your symptoms and ask whether you need help. Most oncologists will not prescribe psychiatric medications except for short-term antianxiety drugs.
- *The oncology nurse.* If your oncologist is unavailable, talk with the head nurse in the oncology office. As a specialist in cancer care, he or she is likely to know a psychiatrist who works well with cancer patients.

- *Your primary care doctor.* The internist, family practitioner, or gyne-cologist you see regularly knows your medical history, can help eval-uate your symptoms, and will make a referral to a psychiatrist if needed.
- *The local hospital's physician referral service.* Most hospitals have a men-tal health program. Even if it doesn't, it can provide you with the names, credentials, and educational backgrounds of psychiatrists in your area. The drawback is that the hospital will recommend only physicians who serve on its staff.
- *Mental health clinics.* Community health clinics supported by tax rev-enues provide services on a sliding scale—the more you make, the more you pay. Who can use such clinics and what services they offer vary from state to state. Find out more by calling your local health department, state health department, or state human services bureau. Alternatively, religious social service agencies such as Catholic Family Service and Jewish Family Service provide mental health services, typi-cally through L.C.S.W.s supervised by a psychologist or psychiatrist. They can also make referrals to outside professionals and thus are good people to ask for the names of qualified psychiatrists.
- *A member of the clergy.* Your minister, priest, or rabbi received training in pastoral counseling in seminary and can assist you in evaluating your need for professional help, as well as provide the names of psychiatrists.
- *A friend or family member who received psychiatric help during cancer treatment.* Ask the friend or family member for the name of the psy-chiatrist he or she worked with. If your friend or family member lives somewhere other than where you do, ask the psychiatrist for a referral to a psychiatric colleague in your area.
- *A self-help patient support group.* If you've made contact with a group offering help to people with cancer, ask other members of the group for the names of psychiatrists they have found helpful.
- *Professional organizations.* The American Psychiatric Association, Can-cer Care, the American Cancer Society, and I Can Cope all provide referrals. See the Resources section in the back of this book for contact information.

CHOOSING A PSYCHIATRIST

Besides the usual credentials of medical school, residency, and a license to practice, a psychiatrist should be certified by the American Board of Psychiatry and Neurology (ABPN). To receive board certification, a psychiatrist must satisfy a series of educational and credentialing criteria and pass extensive written and oral examinations. ABPN certification is not proof of excellence but evidence of clinical competence.

Ideally, too, you should seek out a physician who specializes in consultation-liaison psychiatry or psycho-oncology, the branches of psychiatry that focus on treating the psychiatric problems of the medically ill and those with cancer. Ask the psychiatrist, too, whether he or she has worked before with cancer patients and is comfortable in dealing with the specific problems raised by the disease.

In addition, it is important to select a psychiatrist who fits with you personally. There is more to a beneficial therapeutic relationship than credentials and clinical skill. Since therapy requires the kind of openness and trust between psychiatrist and patient that can develop only when both parties feel comfortable, chemistry is important.

When you are seeking referrals, get the names of two to four candidates. As you talk to the first psychiatrist on the list, pay attention to your emotional reactions. You could be working intimately with this person for many weeks or months or intermittently for years. Does this person have the kind of personal qualities you want? Is he or she on time for the appointment and clearly interested in what you have to say? Does he or she have a sense of humor? Should you encounter difficulties in the evenings or on the weekend, is the psychiatrist or a covering doctor available to you? Is the office setting one in which you feel comfortable? If the match doesn't seem right, try the next physician on your list.

Once you establish a relationship with a psychiatrist during diagnosis, you will probably find that it helps you in dealing with the next round of difficult issues: those raised by treatment—the topic of the next chapter.

5

TREATMENT'S MANY DEMANDS

AFTER THE EMOTIONAL TURMOIL of coming to terms with diagnosis, moving into the treatment phase of cancer may feel like a relief. "Thank God," you say. "At least now I'm *doing* something about this." Yet the desire to begin treatment, and the well-founded optimism that can accompany it, often dissolve upon encountering the realities of surgery, chemotherapy, immunotherapy, hormone therapy, and bone marrow or stem cell transplant. Every form of cancer treatment involves some measure of pain, discomfort, disruption, fatigue, and unpleasantry. Cancer treatment works—but even at its most successful stages, it's still stressful.

The various forms of cancer treatment focus on the body. They aim to seek out, isolate, and destroy cancerous cells. Yet, in a way that underscores the undeniable reality of the mind-body connection, they also affect the emotions, always profoundly and often surprisingly.

So let's look at each of the basic modalities of cancer treatment. After we understand exactly what the treatment is, we will explore the emotional issues commonly associated with it, from the first anticipation of treatment through actually undergoing it.

Surgery

Surgery is the oldest known method of treating cancer. Egyptian medical papyruses dating from 1600 B.C. show physicians cutting tumors out. The lack of anesthesia and the danger of infection, however, hampered surgery until the middle of the nineteenth century, when ether was first used to control pain and sterile technique reduced infection risk. In the century and a half since then, cancer surgery has become increasingly sophisticated and successful, and often less extensive. For example, lumpectomy (removing only the tumor and surrounding breast tissue and some lymph nodes) is now often used for treatment of breast cancer rather than radical mastectomy, which entails taking off the entire breast along with the underlying muscles and lymph nodes.

In modern cancer treatment, surgery can serve to do more than simply remove tumors. Procedures such as laparoscopy and endoscopy—which involve inserting fiber optic devices and small surgical instruments into the body through small incisions or natural passageways such as the esophagus—are used to obtain tissue samples for diagnosis and staging. In advanced disease, surgery plays a role in alleviating symptoms and controlling pain. And reconstructive procedures can be used to rebuild body parts removed in surgery, such as the breast or lower jaw.

Yet, for all the good news from the front, cancer surgery remains difficult and trying for the patient. Knowing what lies ahead, understanding why the surgery is necessary, and being aware of possible methods for handling the stress, pain, and discomfort can help make the surgery as successful as possible.

Facing Surgery

Everyone facing surgery confronts certain basic concerns: a threat to personal invulnerability, worry over entrusting one's life to strangers, trading the familiar environment of family and friends for the institutional setting of the hospital, fear of dying under anesthesia or of going through the surgery partially awake and in pain, and fear about permanent damage to the body. These fears are difficult enough with a relatively simple surgery, such as having a gallbladder removed. But they are vastly heightened in cancer because of the disease's psychological import.

Much of the feeling that surrounds the upcoming surgery focuses on the surgeon. At an unconscious level, most patients deal with the surgeon as they have dealt with other prominent authority figures in their past. Many develop feelings of admiration and affection for surgeons, particularly if they have been well treated by parents, teachers, coaches, members of the clergy, and similar adults when they were children. Others, particularly those who come from abusive or repressive childhoods, can react to surgeons with fear and intimidation or anger and hostility. Being aware of the possibility of this kind of reaction can clear the air and keep the relationship with the surgeon on an even keel.

Knowledge is also an important aspect of preparing yourself for surgery. When you are referred to a surgeon, be sure that the physician making the referral tells you why he or she thinks the operation should be considered as part of your treatment. When you see the surgeon, don't be afraid to ask about the details of the procedure, such as just what will be done, the type of anesthesia that you will receive, the length of time you will spend in the recovery room and hospital, the functions that may be lost temporarily or permanently, and available options for reconstruction or rehabilitation. You may even want to request a specific anesthesiologist. Make sure you talk to the surgeon yourself in order to develop a relationship before the surgery.

In most cases, you also will have a conversation with the anesthesiologist before surgery. This is another opportunity to gain information that can help allay your anxiety. Scientific studies have shown that patients who know how they are going to feel after the operation and what they can do about it experience less pain and use smaller amounts of pain medication than those who are left in the dark. So ask both the anesthesiologist and the surgeon about the type of discomfort you will likely experience after the anesthetic wears off and about the kind of pain control that will be administered during recovery.

Anxiety leading up to surgery is par for the course. In a few people, especially those who have a medical history including panic disorder, generalized anxiety disorder, or a related disorder, this may swell into a preoperative panic so profound that they refuse surgery. In these instances, consultation with a psychiatrist and the possible use of anti-anxiety medication can often provide enormous benefits.

For those experiencing anxiety on a lesser scale, relaxation training before surgery is a great help. Active forms of relation training involve alternately tensing and relaxing major muscle groups, whereas the passive forms are similar to meditation or self-hypnosis. (*Note:* Relaxation techniques are described briefly in Chapter 2. For more information, read the books by Jon Kabat-Zinn and Herbert Benson cited in Sources and Further Reading at the back of this book.)

After Surgery

Waking up in the recovery room immediately after surgery is itself an emotional experience. You are bound to feel helpless and out of control, possibly nauseated from anesthesia, perhaps confused and disoriented. The situation is even more difficult if you are still intubated—that is, if the tube inserted down the trachea (windpipe) to assist in breathing during the operation has been left in place, which is a standard procedure in certain kinds of surgery. If the tube is still in place, you will feel uncomfortable and find talking impossible. After it is removed, you may find your throat sore and your voice husky.

Recovery from any surgery entails at least some degree of pain and discomfort, difficulty in movement, and extreme fatigue. Sometimes this is complicated by feelings of confusion and the loss of cognitive abilities. Patients can lose touch with where they are in space and time or become irritable and agitated, and they may have trouble remembering names or speaking. Called an acute confusional state or delirium, this condition usually arises within the first three or four days after surgery as a result of adverse reactions to anesthesia or medication or because of metabolic imbalances in the body. Delirium can also strike alcoholics who are withdrawing from alcohol. Confusion is particularly likely to occur in the elderly, who react more strongly to changes in their daily routines and to the stress of an unfamiliar environment than do younger people. Such delirium can be controlled with medication and support, and it usually lasts no more than a week, with the full recovery of all cognitive functions sometimes taking longer.

Recovering from surgery can bring on a low, or depressed, mood. This may in part be the result of commonly used narcotic or opiate pain medications, which are highly effective against pain but can affect mood, as well as cause nausea and constipation. This low mood has the potential to grow into a significant depression, particularly in cases where the surgery is extensive, such as amputation of a limb because of bone cancer; where the procedure can produce infertility or sexual dysfunction; or where the tumor is found to be larger than suspected and prospects for full recovery are less optimistic. Faced with adapting to a new style of life, such patients go through a period of shock, followed by emotional turmoil that can lead to major depression accompanied by thoughts of suicide. Statements such as, "My life is over. What do I have to live for?" and "There's no reason to put my family through any more pain," are common.

If depressed mood overwhelms you, seek support from your family and friends. Distraction helps, too. That is, do things you enjoy that remove you from your feelings a little bit. For some people, it's classical music; for others, it's funny movies. But if these coping mechanisms fail to resolve your low mood, and particularly if thoughts about self-destruction continue, consultation with a psychiatrist, especially one with training in psycho-oncology, is the best solution.

The Pain Question

Even under the best of circumstances, surgery hurts. The pain that inevitably follows a surgical procedure can bring up emotional reactions based on one's experiences, value systems, and psychological makeup.

Some patients, particularly men, see postsurgical pain as a proving ground for machismo. Lou, a sixty-year-old construction worker who had grown up on the Bronx's mean streets, was one of those. He had been a tough guy from the time he was a toddler, and he had spent his life working in a world where admitting pain was viewed as a sign of weakness. When I met Lou, he had undergone colon surgery for a cancerous tumor two days earlier. Recovery from abdominal surgery is always unpleasant, and removing a segment of intestine produces painful cramps. Lou was obviously in pain. He was sweating and restless, and he kept grabbing the sheets in his sweaty fists and clenching his teeth as we spoke. Yet Lou had refused the pain medication his surgeon had prescribed.

"That stuff's for sissies," he told me. "If any of my work buddies saw me taking those fancy drugs, they'd bust me in the chops."

I looked around the room. "I don't see any of them here," I said. "And I won't tell if you won't."

Lou gave me a look to kill.

"Look, this isn't about your willpower or toughness, which you obviously have in spades," I continued. "It's about good medicine." I went on to explain to Lou that the pain was slowing his recovery. With the body focusing on the painful sensations in his abdomen, it didn't have the wherewithal to heal from surgery.

"You mean I can get back to work faster if I take pain medication?" Lou said.

I nodded.

"You're on," he said.

Within fifteen minutes of his first dose of morphine, Lou was resting much more comfortably. And, in fact, his recovery went much better from then on.

Unfortunately, it sometimes happens that a physician is insensitive to a patient's pain. I ran into this situation when a surgeon asked me to evaluate a forty-five-year-old patient named Marsha who had undergone partial removal of a lung for a cancerous mass. She was, the doctor told me, an actress and "just what you'd suspect—demanding, overwrought. Hysterical if you ask me." Yet when I met Marsha, she seemed more beleaguered and frightened than dramatic. She was clearly suffering significant pain.

"You're hurting, aren't you?" I said.

She nodded. The pain made the movement of her head weak, almost desperate.

"What happens when you tell your doctor about it?"

She gave me a wry smile. "He says, 'Hang in there.' Fat lot of good that does me." Marsha explained that she had tried to tell the medical staff how bad she felt, but she had gotten nowhere. I could tell that the pain confused and weakened her so much that it was difficult for her to advocate for herself. So her complaints had gone unheard.

A review of Marsha's medical chart made it clear to me that she was being undermedicated. I let her know that I would talk to her doctor. As politely and gently as possible, I raised the issue with the surgeon, who had somehow gotten into a power struggle with Marsha. He increased the dose of medication, and Marsha's pain dropped into the zone of tolerability.

Pain in cancer is inescapable. Still, given today's medical technology, there is no need for significant suffering. Pain control following surgery actually makes for faster recovery. And if sleep is difficult or anxiety is prominent, the temporary use of a medication will often solve the problem. If you are hurting intolerably, physically or emotionally, advocate for yourself or have a friend or family member speak up for you.

Emotions That Arise Based on the Kind of Surgery

Following surgery, specific emotional issues can arise that are related to the site of the operation and the type of procedure.

COLON

In most early-stage tumors of the large intestine, a section can be removed and the remaining portions rejoined to allow normal bowel function. But in some more advanced cases and in tumors involving the rectum, all or most of the large intestine has to be excised, making a colostomy necessary. An opening, or stoma, is created in the front of the abdomen and the end of the intestine is attached to it. A bag secured to the stoma catches fecal material, or, alternatively, a reservoir is created inside the body and is emptied of waste by inserting a tube through the stoma. In some cases, after healing is complete, the surgery is reversed and the bowel is reconnected.

When I saw my first colostomy in medical school, I was shocked and upset. It was disturbing to see what is normally on the inside of the body moved to the outside. And given the equation of feces with dirt and filth, the surgery struck me as terribly unclean.

Many patients who receive a colostomy feel the same way—palpably dirtied and mutilated. Disgust, embarrassment, anger, and shame arise from having this kind of wound. These feelings worsen as the patient deals with learning how to care for the stoma day to day and may lead to depression, chronic anxiety, and social isolation as the individual hesitates to leave home for fear of an embarrassing accident. Feeling mutilated and unattractive, colostomy patients often hesitate to be sexual with their partners, adding to their isolation and creating stress in their intimate relationships.

Some colostomy patients are able to resolve many of these issues with the help of friends and family. But in a significant number, the psychological issues remain well after surgery and recovery and should be addressed with professional help.

BREAST

The breast carries such a multitude of sexual and maternal meanings that surgery for breast cancer is bound to have major emotional import on the patient. Depression, anxiety, and low self-esteem are common reactions, whether a woman undergoes a mastectomy (complete removal of the breast) or a lumpectomy (removal of the tumor and the surrounding tissue only, with the remainder of the breast left in place). The psychological consequences of the two surgeries are largely the same, except that lumpectomy patients suffer less disturbance of their body image than do mastectomy patients. Reconstructive surgery—in which the breast mound is rebuilt with a saline implant or tissue transplanted from elsewhere in the woman's body—can help restore a more normal body sense. Most women who have had such reconstruction feel that it helped in their psychological recovery from the cancer.

While breast surgery carries powerful emotional repercussions involving sexuality and reproduction for women of all ages, they are most poignant among younger women of childbearing age. Ally, a thirty-eight-year-old married mother of two, came to me for what she described as "marital strain." She was a tall woman, clearly attractive, but she hid her body under layers of baggy clothes. She had been through a lot. About a year earlier, she had undergone removal of both her breasts for cancer, followed by six months of chemotherapy. Recently, she had had reconstructive surgery with saline implants.

"The strange thing is that Michael"—Ally's husband—"and I were so together and connected through the entire process," she explained. "All the way through the surgeries and the chemo, he was my biggest supporter and my best friend. Now that things are getting back to something like normal, he wants to make love. And I don't. I just don't have any sexual feelings toward him." She shrugged. "It's not him. I don't have sexual feelings toward anyone."

"How is this affecting your marriage?" I asked.

"There's this before-the-storm silence in the air. Then, when we try to talk about it, I get all uptight and Michael turns angry and withdraws. He even accused me of not loving him. That's crazy. It's just that things are different." Ally's eyes filled with tears.

Before the cancer, Ally and Michael had a sex life she described as "fantastic." Cancer changed how she felt about her body.

"I was always comfortable with my femininity," she related. "Cancer treatment changed that. My breasts became foreign to me. They were a source of fear and worry, objects to be probed, to have needles stuck in them. Finally, they were cut off, and I came out of surgery feeling . . . well, mutilated. Now, even with my breasts reconstructed, I feel like a poor excuse for who I used to be. I feel different, unattractive, unfeminine, damaged. How could I be attractive to anyone, especially Michael? He knows what the real me used to feel and look like."

Ally had a clear handle on where her difficulty had arisen. Overwhelmed by the changes in her body, she literally didn't know who she was. She needed to discover her body again, to grow beyond the emotional and physical pain of her disease. I suggested that she and Michael see a therapist who could help them learn ways to communicate their concerns and to reconnect in terms of intimacy, love, and sexuality. Such treatment is a combination of marital and sex therapy. The psychotherapist they saw created a safe environment in which Ally and Michael were able to understand their unhealthy communication patterns and adopt new ways to express their feelings. Once they reconnected emotionally, their therapist incorporated some behavioral techniques to reestablish their sexual intimacy. Such techniques include "homework assignments"—learning to pleasure each other in nonerogenous areas, then resuming sexual contact after trust and comfort have developed. For Michael and Ally, as well as for many other couples who have been through similar experiences, this therapeutic approach worked.

GENITOURINARY

Like cancer of the breast, malignant disease in the genital and urinary organs—primarily the *prostate, bladder,* and *testicles* in men, and the *uterus, cervix, bladder,* and *ovaries* in women—can have major sexual implications. Both the disease and the treatment can either dampen desire or alter sexual responsiveness and capacity. Some of the effects are physical—for example, cutting the nerves leading to the genitals affects sexual performance. In addition, the psychological implications of surgery for genitourinary cancer can be profound.

Barry, a forty-year-old history teacher, was referred to me by his oncologist for erectile dysfunction—that is, impotence, or the inability to achieve or sustain an erection. About six months earlier, Barry had noticed a hard spot in one testicle, which was determined to be cancerous. That testicle was removed, while the healthy one was left in place. Barry then underwent a course of chemotherapy, a standard procedure for the type of cancer he had. Although his healthy testicle was, after several months, able to produce more than enough testosterone to support even the most vigorous sex life, Barry was now unable to get an erection.

Barry said to me in his no-nonsense style, "I know it's all in my head. I just can't figure out what *it* is."

After he described the ordeal of surgery and chemotherapy, I asked him what treatment had felt like.

"It stunk. I got castrated. Truth is, I just don't feel like much of a man anymore." Barry's voice was self-conscious, tinged with shame.

I acknowledged Barry's feelings and asked him to tell me about his past, particularly the experiences that created his sense of manhood. He told me he was the youngest of three sons, born to a father who operated a bar in their blue-collar hometown and sat on the city council. It was the kind of place where tackle football was played without helmets and men drank their whisky straight.

"Who you were was a function of home runs, touchdowns, and sexual conquests." Barry said. "I know now it was all a lot of male chauvinistic nonsense, but it sure shaped who I am."

This understanding provided an opening. I suggested to Barry that we work together to untangle his sometimes-distorted feelings about manhood and broaden his view of what the male gender was about. He agreed. Within a few months, his sexuality was back on track. And he became more capable of intimate relationships with women, both as friends and lovers.

Treatment for prostate cancer also entails at least some change in sexuality. Thankfully, new nerve-sparing surgical techniques reduce the likelihood of postsurgical erectile dysfunction. However, removal of the prostate and adjacent tissues, which store most of the semen, means that little or no fluid is ejaculated at orgasm—a change that can be disconcerting. For men who suffer from erectile dysfunction following surgery or radiation, drugs such as Viagra, vacuum pumps, and penile implants can prove helpful, along with counseling with a psychotherapist skilled in marital and sexual issues.

Similar sexual problems can arise in women who have had radical cancer surgery or radiation of the pelvis. Changes to the vagina and vulva may make intercourse difficult or painful, and the hormones that influence sexual response may be lost if the ovaries are removed. In addition, since body image greatly influences how women perceive themselves, the removal of the uterus or ovaries and the loss of the ability to procreate can be devastating, particularly to a young woman. A number of solutions are possible. Lubricants may help with sex, as can consultation with a sex therapist, who may be able to help a couple discover new avenues of lovemaking. Hormone replacement therapy can make up for the loss of the ovaries if the cancer is not hormone-dependent. Women who are mourning the loss of their fertility can be encouraged to seek other ways of being maternal, such as adopting children or committing themselves to work with children. In all cases, education, support, and psychotherapy during recovery are key.

HEAD AND NECK

Disfigurement and facial mutilation are the key issues in cancers of the head and neck. A lost breast can be replaced with a prosthesis, a colostomy can be covered with clothing, but a surgically altered face cannot be concealed. Attractiveness, the ability to succeed socially, and the expression of emotions all depend on the face. Altering or removing the features strikes a strong blow at self-identity. In addition, the patient may have to deal with impaired or lost speech, taste, or smell. Experiencing depression and anxiety is common among such patients.

Lindsay, a twenty-six-year-old graduate student, had been referred to me because she had become agoraphobic (fearful of crowded public spaces) and withdrawn, often missing classes and jeopardizing her progress toward an advanced degree. Recently, she had completed surgery and radiation for a localized cancer in her left lower jaw. When she came into the consultation room, she was careful to keep the right side of her face turned to me. At first withdrawn, even sullen, she slowly opened up.

"I feel like the Phantom of the Opera, but without the mask and the music," she explained. "I look like a freak. People just stare at me and turn away. I used to look okay, but now I'm just plain ugly."

The truth of the matter was that Lindsay was cute and her jaw reconstruction was remarkable. Nothing could be seen except for a slight indentation on her left jaw and a small scar. She looked a long way from monstrous. Yet when I told her that, she shook her head. "I don't know you and I don't trust you," she said. "There's no reason for me to believe you."

As Lindsay and I worked together—and as she came to know and trust me—we discovered that she had always fallen short of her expected view of herself. All through her life, she had felt she was never pretty enough, tall enough, thin enough, smart enough, and so on. She had constantly tried to improve her physical self, which she considered more important than her internal assets: her obvious intelligence, kindness, and quick, gentle wit.

We also discovered that Lindsay was a world-class projector—that is, she unconsciously assumed that others had the same negative thoughts about her that she had about herself. She came to realize that no one saw her as a freak. In the end, Lindsay came to perceive herself as less than perfect—aren't we all?—but as a person of value and worth, anyway.

A similar journey is to be found in Lucy Grealy's *Autobiography of a Face*. Now an accomplished poet, writer, and teacher, Grealy lost much of her jaw to cancer during childhood and endured a long series of reconstructive surgeries. The autobiographic story of her journey toward self-acceptance is powerful and moving, and you may wish to read it to gain a new perspective on yourself and your situation.

Radiation

Radiation plays a number of roles in cancer treatment. It is used as the primary therapy for Hodgkin's disease and throat cancer and is an option for localized prostate cancer. Radiation is also combined with surgery, chemotherapy, or both in treating breast cancer, connective-tissue cancers (sarcomas), lung cancer, and cervical cancer. In advanced disease, radiation is used to shrink tumors and reduce pain and other symptoms.

The reason why radiation works in treating cancer arises in the intersection of cell biology and physics. When high-dose X-rays strike living tissue, they raise the molecules in that tissue to an unstable, ionized state. This reaction disrupts the chemical bonds holding together DNA (deoxyribonucleic acid—the cell's genetic material), proteins, and other cell components. Cells that are dividing rapidly, such as cancer cells, are most sensitive to this potentially lethal reaction. Cells that are dividing less quickly, such as those in nerve and muscle tissue, are affected much less and recover from the radiation more quickly. Thus, radiation selectively kills cancer cells while causing less damage to surrounding normal tissue. In recent years, radiation oncologists and their equipment have become increasingly skilled at targeting cancerous tumors and sparing healthy tissues and organs.

Radiation treatments are delivered in two basic ways. In teletherapy, or external beam radiation, the radiation source lies outside the body. Aimed at achieving a cancer remission, radiation treatment is usually given Monday through Friday for six weeks. When the purpose of teletherapy is only to shrink a tumor or reduce pain or symptoms (so-called palliative treatment), the radiation is given five days a week for two weeks. In brachytherapy, the radiation source is inserted temporarily into the patient's body in a surgical procedure, and then the patient is isolated for several days. At the end of this period, the radiation source is removed, although low-energy radiation sources called seeds are occasionally left permanently in the tumor. Brachytherapy is now being used to treat localized prostate cancer, since it causes fewer side effects than teletherapy or surgical removal of the prostate.

Hiroshima, Side Effects, and Emotions

At first glance, radiation therapy looks like a lark compared to surgery. There's no general anesthesia to worry about, no painful incision to recover from. But radiation has a downside that plays into emotional reactions to the therapy.

The highly technological nature of radiation treatment and the large machines used in this therapy often cause significant fear and apprehension. Small tattoos are placed on the body to guide the radiation beam; some people find them to be visible reminders of their disease, something like an oncological scarlet letter or mark of Cain. The need for isolation in brachytherapy often feels like solitary confinement to those patients receiving it. And finally there is fear of radiation; after all, the beam being directed against the cancer is a first cousin to the powerful explosive that flattened Hiroshima and Nagasaki and condemned tens of thousands of people to lingering death from radiation sickness. That thought, while lying under a radiological apparatus, can lead to a certain disquiet.

Then there are the side effects of treatment. Localized burning and pain are to be expected. An all-over fatigue and an increased need to sleep arise from the body's response to the cell damage caused by radiation. Nausea is common when the whole body, the upper half of the body, or the lower abdomen is irradiated (but less likely in radiation of the chest, upper abdomen, pelvis, head, and neck). Radiation of the head may cause swelling of the brain, which can cause a variety of symptoms (headache, confusion, and mood changes, such as irritability) and the need for counteracting medication. Full-blown radiation sickness, characterized by significant nausea, vomiting, and hair loss, is rare, but it does sometimes happen. It may even be life-threatening, but it is very treatable.

Most of these side effects improve after radiation ends, but certain ones may continue or even arise well after therapy. These include changes in the lungs that make breathing difficult during exercise, retarded growth in children, and abnormally low thyroid activity. Radiation for head and neck cancer sometimes causes changes in taste and a very dry mouth, which may lead to poor nutrition and to dental problems. Persistent diarrhea may result from abdominal radiation. And both sterility and sexual dysfunction may result from radiation treatment of cancer in the genital or urinary systems. Fortunately, most of these complications can be well managed.

Experiencing Helplessness and Depression After Radiation

I have come to call it the *Star Wars* syndrome: Often the radiation patient feels passive, zapped, and powerless. As a result, radiation therapy can have profound psychological effects, particularly for those who are used to being in control.

Peter, a sixty-year-old businessman who had been known for his energy and enthusiasm, was referred to me by his oncologist after Peter's wife had reported that he was withdrawn, refusing to go to work or engage in family or social life, and neither sleeping nor eating. Formerly a clotheshorse, Peter was now sitting around the house unshaven, wearing sweat pants and an old Yankees T-shirt. Although he dressed up a bit to come see me, the expensive European suit looked two sizes too large and he had forgotten his tie. The gray stubble covering his face said that he still hadn't shaved. Peter's eyes were dull and lifeless, and when I said hello, he answered in a flat voice.

I knew our initial moments would be difficult. After the usual social pleasantries, I asked, "So, how do you feel about coming to speak to me?"

"Don't care," he said. "I've seen so many doctors in the past three months that seeing another doesn't make any difference. I'm numb to it all. So I'm seeing you; no big deal."

Despite his surface apathy, Peter was willing to tell me his story. A few months earlier, he had gone in for a routine yearly physical. The standard blood work revealed a sudden rise in his prostate-specific antigen (PSA) level, a finding that can signal prostate cancer. Peter's physician referred him to a urologist, who performed an ultrasound scan of the prostate and a biopsy, and, after additional tests, diagnosed Peter with early-stage, localized prostate cancer. After weighing the pros and cons of surgery versus radiation, Peter had chosen radiation. When I saw him, he had completed about half the treatment and was tolerating the therapy well.

"How did you find out you have prostate cancer?" I asked. "And how did it feel when you found out?"

"My urologist called me at work," Peter answered. "When he told me that I had cancer, I didn't really feel anything. I haven't felt anything yet."

"How would you describe your mood these days?"

"Either I don't care, or I want to be left alone."

"But what happens in the middle of the night, when you're all alone with your thoughts? What do you think about then?"

For the first time, Peter made eye contact with me. Small tears formed along his lower lids. "I don't sleep much. All I can think about is there's this big thing in my life I can't control. No matter how hard I try, my efforts are worthless. I have to be passive. I have to let other people take care of me."

Beginning radiation—with the need to lie flat and still under a huge machine five days a week—exacerbated this feeling. As the therapy began, Peter slipped slowly into a flat, low mood. He found it difficult to sleep, lost his appetite, and found no pleasure in the things that had once turned him on—like following the Yankees, playing tennis with his young adult sons, reading contemporary fiction, and exploring ethnic restaurants with his wife. He had not considered suicide, but he admitted that deep into his sleepless nights his thoughts turned to "just not being; what it feels like to enter the darkness and stay there."

Peter was experiencing a classic major depressive episode. In a way, that was surprising; he had an excellent prognosis, with a highly treatable form of cancer, and the prospect of many more years of life. Why, then, was Peter's reaction so profound?

"It's ironic," he said. "It's not the cancer itself that's got me down. It's my sense of emotional weakness and the loss of control."

"You sound as if you have failed," I said.

He was quiet for a moment. "You're right," he said. "I feel as if I have failed. *I'm* not taking care. I'm the one being taken care of. To me, that's failure."

The eldest child in his family, Peter had become the effective head of the household in high school, when his father died of lung cancer. He took care of his mother and his three siblings, working and going to school simultaneously. Later, he carried that way of being over into his own family; he judged his self-worth by how well he cared for his wife and children.

Then cancer and radiation therapy had turned Peter into a passive recipient. As the emotional tables were turned, Peter tumbled into depression.

Fortunately, Peter's emotional disorder was as treatable as his cancer. I prescribed antidepressants plus a brief course of sleep medication to help him rest. And over several months of psychotherapy, we discussed the value of allowing oneself to be cared for. As Peter came to understand that he was a man of value and worth even when he was lying helpless under a radiation machine, his low mood began to lift.

Standard Chemotherapy, Hormonal Therapy, and Immunotherapy

Oncologists now have access to a wide variety of cancer medications and they use them in an equally wide variety of combinations, both alone and in concert with surgery or radiation. Standard chemotherapy agents selectively attack fast-dividing cancer cells, but they can also affect normal tissues with fast-dividing cells such as hair follicles, bone marrow, and the lining of the mouth and intestine. Hormone therapy medications are used against cancers that are hormone-responsive. For example, advanced metastasized prostate cancer grows rapidly in the presence of the male hormone testosterone. Suppressing testosterone production and administering medications that mimic female hormones slows the progression of the disease. Tamoxifen has become a widely used treatment against certain kinds of breast cancer because it blocks the female hormone estrogen. Hormonal treatments are also employed against certain uterine cancers, leukemia, and lymphoma. Immunotherapy treatments work by bolstering the body's natural immune system and increase its ability to combat the cancer. Ongoing research in producing anticancer vaccines offers the prospect of reducing side effects and improving effectiveness. In these still-experimental therapies, tumor tissue is removed surgically, then used to create a vaccine that is injected back into the patient. The patient's immune system now registers the cancer as foreign and attacks it as it would any outside invader.

Standard chemotherapy, hormone therapy, and immunotherapy all can have unpleasant side effects. Best known for causing vomiting and hair loss, standard chemotherapy may also reduce immunity against infection by suppressing bone marrow. Hormone therapy, likewise, has undesirable side effects. Female hormones feminize the male body, for example, decreasing muscle mass and sexual drive and leading to weight gain and breast swelling. Tamoxifen causes premature menopause, complete with hot flashes. As for immunotherapy, it too can cause unpleasant side effects, such as overall flu-like symptoms.

Fortunately, excellent antidotes exist to control the side effects of cancer medications. For example, a new class of drugs, which includes Kytril and Zofran, is extremely effective against nausea and vomiting. Relaxation techniques such as meditation and hypnosis have been specifically adapted to minimize the flu-like symptoms and fatigue that accompany chemical treatment.

The following tables list the most common cancer medications (brand names first, with generic names in parentheses) and their possible side effects.

Standard Chemotherapy Agents and Their Side Effects

Standard Chemotherapy Agents	Side Effects
Adriamycin (doxorubicin)	nausea and vomiting, bone marrow suppression, red urine (harmless), hair loss
Blenoxane (bleomycin)	occasional allergic reaction, fever, rash or brown skin discoloration
Carboplatin (paraplatin)	nausea (usually mild), bone marrow suppression, hearing difficulty in upper range
Cytoxan (cyclophosphamide)	bone marrow suppression, nausea and vomiting, hair loss, bladder irritation
Fludara (fludarabine)	bone marrow suppression, nausea, diarrhea, mouth soreness, coughing or breathing problems, confusion
Gemzar (gemcytobine)	nausea, diarrhea, mouth soreness, bone marrow suppression, fever, skin rash, flu-like symptoms, mild hair loss
Idamycin (idarubicin)	bone marrow suppression, hair loss, nausea and vomiting, mouth soreness, diarrhea
Leucovorin (folinic acid)	mouth soreness, diarrhea, skin irritation, and bone marrow suppression
Leukeran (chlorambucil)	bone marrow suppression
Matulane (procarbazine)	bone marrow suppression, nausea and vomiting, flushing if taken with alcohol or certain foods including cheese
Mutamycin (mitomycin-C)	nausea and vomiting, bone marrow suppression
Oncovin (vincristine)	nausea and vomiting, mild hair loss, numb fingers and toes, constipation
Platinol (cisplatin)	nausea and vomiting; numbness, tingling, or weakness in hands and feet; bone marrow suppression
Taxol (paclitaxel)	bone marrow suppression, nausea, diarrhea, sore mouth, hair loss, fatigue, slowed heart rate
Vepesid (etoposide, VP-16)	bone marrow suppression, nausea, mouth sores

Immunotherapy Agents and Their Side Effects

Immunotherapy Agents	Side Effects
Aldesleukin, Proleukin (interleukin-2)	nausea, vomiting, confusion, fever, chills, low blood pressure, bone marrow suppression, depressed mood
Intron, Roferon (interferon)	fatigue, fever, muscle aches and pain, depression, possible bone marrow suppression
Rituxan (rituximab, anti-CD20 antibody)	chills, fever (rarely), wheezing or low blood pressure

Hormonal Agents and Their Side Effects

Hormonal Agents	Side Effects
Arimidex (anastrozole)	hot flashes, vaginal bleeding, vaginal discharge and dryness, irregular periods, depression, dizziness, leg cramps, hair thinning, confusion, fatigue, weight gain
Deltasone (prednisone)	water retention, heartburn, difficulty sleeping, mood changes including anxiety, depression, irritability, or inappropriate elation (hypomania), increased appetite with weight gain (combining medication with food or antacids prevents some side effects)
Lupron (leuprolide)	nausea, hot flashes, erectile dysfunction, breast swelling
Megace (megestrol)	fluid retention, hot flashes, weight gain
Nolvadex (tamoxifen)	hot flashes, vaginal bleeding, vaginal discharge and dryness, irregular periods, depression, dizziness, leg cramps, hair thinning, confusion, fatigue, weight gain

The Emotional Side of Chemotherapy

At first, chemotherapy can seem almost easy, despite the emotional distress that invariably accompanies cancer. Typically, you go to the infusion clinic and sit in a large, comfortable chair while a nurse hooks up an IV to put the medication into one of your veins. Usually the procedure is no more than minimally uncomfortable, and an hour or two later you go home. Normally the first session is not noteworthy. Then the side effects begin to worsen with each treatment and chemotherapy turns into an ordeal. Many patients say it becomes harder and harder to show up for treatment, yet they are afraid to quit, fearing that stopping therapy too soon tips the odds in the cancer's favor. So they continue reluctantly. Knowing what to expect, and understanding what to do about it, can help you get through the treatment cycle. So here's what you may experience:

- *Hair loss.* Many chemotherapeutic agents cause some or all of the hair to fall out. Almost universally, patients find this upsetting; the sudden baldness strikes a blow at self-identity. Some men respond by shaving their heads and wearing a hat. Women, however, who are often defined by their hair and put a great deal of energy into its care, suffer more greatly from the baldness. It helps to remember that your hair *will* grow back after treatment—albeit slowly and differently (usually more curly) than it was before, but it eventually returns to the way it was. In the interim, excellent wigs are available.

- *Anticipatory nausea.* Nausea and vomiting are common side effects of chemotherapy and some immunotherapy agents. Because the patient learns that nausea is a likely outcome of treatment, a classical Pavlovian condition can occur here. Pavlov, you may remember, was the early twentieth-century Russian physiologist who conditioned dogs to salivate involuntarily when he rang a bell. First, he sounded the bell when he fed the dogs, causing them to salivate in anticipation of the meal. Later, when he rang the bell without feeding the dogs, the animals salivated anyway. They had been conditioned to associate the bell with food, and salivation was their involuntary response. Much the same thing can happen with the nausea following chemotherapy. Knowing what is likely to happen, the patient becomes nauseous and starts vomiting even before the medication is infused.

   A thirty-five-year-old college administrator, Marlene, was suffering from non-Hodgkin's lymphoma, a cancer treated primarily with chemotherapy. Although she was given antinausea medications, they proved insufficient to stop the vomiting that plagued Marlene after each weekly treatment. Within a few months, the anxiety she felt before treatment turned into a round of anticipatory nausea and vomiting. Just the simple thought of the infusion clinic would turn Marlene's stomach and send her running to the bathroom. Soon, the picture of a hospital room on television or a single whiff of medicinal alcohol was enough to trigger vomiting. The experience was so upsetting that Marlene missed two consecutive chemotherapy sessions.

Fortunately, the infusion nurse knew what was happening and referred Marlene to me. After learning a series of relaxation techniques and undergoing hypnosis by a well-trained practitioner, Marlene broke the link between her anticipation and the nausea. She completed therapy without any more anticipatory reactions and with only modest discomfort following each treatment.

- *Fatigue*. Chemotherapy commonly produces a constant feeling of exhaustion that makes it hard to complete the ordinary tasks of day-to-day life. Some people adapt relatively easily to this reality. For others, though, the fatigue is difficult to handle. The difference has a great deal to do with personality style and psychological makeup.

Anna, a forty-five-year-old Roman Catholic mother of six and a horse breeder by profession, had been diagnosed with a rare blood cell cancer. The good news was that the disease was treatable; the bad news was that treatment consisted of chemotherapy infusions every few weeks for several years. Although optimistic about a positive outcome, Anna came to see me because she had gradually become frustrated and depressed as the treatment progressed.

On the very first visit to my office, Anna plopped herself down in a chair by my desk, sighed, and said, "I'm so tired."

Given that the fatigue was to be expected from a long-term chemotherapy regimen such as the one Anna was undergoing, I wondered why the fatigue upset her so.

She knew why. "I can't be the mother I should be to my children," she said. "That's my most important job, and I just can't do it like I should."

As we spoke further, I noticed that Anna used the word *should* again and again. It was a driving word in her personal vocabulary—but with her psychological history, that wasn't surprising. The eldest of four siblings and the only daughter, Anna served as stand-in mom to her brothers, since their own mother had chronic cardiac disease that eventually made her completely bedridden. Trained to be responsible for everything as an adolescent surrogate parent, Anna was consumed by guilt when her brothers were getting less than what she saw as proper care. She carried this attitude over into her own mothering. Until her cancer diagnosis, she had been a super-mom, the kind who ran her own business, carted the kids to every athletic event, helped out in the classroom at the parochial school, and still found time to bake cookies. Now, because of the chemotherapy, she simply couldn't keep up with that style of life any longer. Yet, rather than give herself the room to be tired and sick, she judged herself harshly.

With a period of brief psychotherapy, Anna gained insight into the way she punished herself, and she learned how to become more accepting. Soon she said *should* much less, and she was able to approach her disease and the rest of her life with greater acceptance and equanimity.

There are excellent medications available that can help overcome fatigue. With proper medical supervision, they can stimulate without becoming habit-forming.

• *Confusion and delirium.* As we read earlier, the state of profound confusion called delirium can occur after surgery. It may also arise as a reaction to certain chemotherapy medications, which are toxic to the central nervous system. Delirium, which is characterized by disorientation and the inability to sustain attention, and may also be accompanied by false perceptions (hallucinations) and untrue beliefs (delusions), is very frightening for the patient. Fortunately, it is temporary and can be controlled.

When I walked into his hospital room, Chester, a fifty-two-year-old undergoing aggressive chemotherapy for acute leukemia, turned to me and said, "Who the hell are you, soldier, and what do you want?"

"I'm not a soldier. I'm Dr. Granet, and you're in the hospital." I spoke firmly and clearly, in hope of reorienting Chester to the reality he had lost.

"As if I care!" he said. "Can't you hear the choppers outside? This is Vietnam; there's a war going on. Stay alert or you could be dead meat." Chester was right about the choppers: His room was near the landing pad where helicopters transporting emergency patients landed. But the noise working on his delusional mind had taken him back to his tour as an infantry squad leader in Vietnam over thirty years ago.

I prescribed a small amount of a tranquilizer, which reduced his agitation and confusion. The nurses and I kept reminding Chester that he was in New York, not Vietnam, and no war was being fought. We put a clock in his room to tell him the correct time, left the lights on to alleviate fear, and had a family member stay with him day and night. Within two days, Chester had become calm and once again oriented to reality.

Bone Marrow and Stem Cell . Transplantation

Bone marrow and peripheral blood stem cell transplants may qualify as the most rigorous and difficult cancer treatments. Even the therapeutic rationale behind them is demanding. Basically, the patient is given doses of radiation, chemotherapy, or both so severe that they could be lethal. Then, before the patient succumbs, he or she is "rescued" with infusions of the same kind of blood precursor cells that have been killed off by radiation and chemotherapy. The patient develops a new complement of cancer-free blood cells and a renovated immune system as he or she recovers.

Bone marrow and stem cell transplants are effective against certain leukemias and lymphomas, Hodgkin's disease, small-cell lung cancer, multiple myeloma (a bone cancer), advanced ovarian and testicular cancer, and sarcomas (connective tissue cancers). Although they have been used against breast cancer, recent research shows they may be no more effective in that disease than standard radiation and chemotherapy.

Some bone marrow transplant patients receive the marrow from a genetically similar donor—ideally, an identical twin—but most patients both donate and receive their own marrow. With the patient anesthetized, the marrow—which is the blood cell–producing tissue in the hollow center of bones—is drawn out with a vacuum pump, then treated to kill any cancer cells it contains. After the patient recovers from the surgery, he or she is subjected to extremely high doses of chemotherapy, radiation, or both over three to ten days. This approach is more lethal to cancer cells than the smaller doses used in standard treatment, but it also proves highly toxic to the patient. At this point, the cleansed marrow cells are infused into the patient's bloodstream, providing a new source of healthy cells.

Peripheral blood stem cell transplants are similar in some ways. Instead of undergoing surgery to remove bone marrow, however, blood is taken from the patient, and the blood cell precursors known as stem cells are removed and collected. The stem cells are then injected into the patient after high-dose chemotherapy, radiation, or both. Autologous stem cell therapy—that is, the cells come from the patient—is easier on the patient, in part because there is no surgery to remove marrow and no risk of the body rejecting the transplant since it is the patient's own tissue. In addition, it is currently less expensive than allogenic (donor) transplants.

In both kinds of transplants, the period following the procedure is very difficult. Because of the pretransplant treatment, the patient is typically suffering from hair loss, severe nausea, diarrhea, painful mouth sores, and lack of appetite. Less often, there are malfunctions of the heart, lungs, liver, or kidneys. The mouth sores, nausea, and diarrhea can be so bad that the patient cannot eat, necessitating total intravenous nutrition until the digestive system can heal enough to tolerate food.

Most significantly, the bone marrow or stem cell transplant patient has practically no working immune system. It takes two to four weeks for the first new blood cells to arise from the transplanted tissue, and up to several months for the entire immune system to regenerate. Some patients undergoing stem cell transplants may recover more quickly. Still, during the first several weeks after transplantation, the patient is highly vulnerable to any passing infection. Even an ordinary cold can prove fatal. As a precaution against infection, the patient is kept in protective isolation, confined to a small area and required to wear a face mask and latex gloves when outside it. Special filters protect the airflow in the room against bacterial contamination. Medical staff and visitors have to scrub their hands before entering the room, and may be required to put on a surgical gown and mask. Patients are kept in isolation until their blood count reaches a certain safety point, which can take from two weeks to several months, depending on a variety of factors. Even after discharge, the patient is medically unstable and has to be monitored regularly in an outpatient setting. Fatigue and weakness can persist for six to twelve months after treatment.

Bone marrow and peripheral blood stem cell transplants have profound effects on the emotions. Research has found that before treatment, many patients selectively block out threatening information about the procedure. In a way, this makes sense as a way of coping with a difficult therapy, particularly for those whose only hope for survival lies in bone marrow or stem cell transplantation. Then there are the severe side effects of the chemotherapy or radiation, which are very taxing. Isolation during recovery also takes a toll. Even though it protects the patient, he or she may feel like an outcast. Hospital discharge, while eagerly anticipated by the patient, is also a crisis. As the security blanket is withdrawn, anxiety rises. "What if something goes wrong?" the patient asks. "Without a nurse right around the corner, what am I going to do when there's a problem?" And once the patient is out of the hospital, he or she faces a regimen of self-care practices and rules necessary to guard against infection until the new immune system is working fully. Given the long, hard road the transplant patient has traveled, returning to normal life is itself a demanding task. However, since much is now understood about the emotional reactions to transplantation, psychological intervention provides great comfort.

The enormity of such reactions was illustrated dramatically in Vince, a fifty-four-year-old internist. He understood bone marrow transplants intellectually but found himself staggered by the emotional and physical toll of the therapy when he went through it for myeloma (a plasma cell cancer). I saw him six months after his successful transplant was completed.

Vince explained why he came in for a consultation. "My family and colleagues think since I'm a doc, I should be up and fully functioning now that it's been six months. But, I tell you, it's been like a war from the beginning. First the diagnosis, with one test after another, then the bone marrow harvest, then the chemo. I was physically ill in a way I couldn't remember since having the flu as a kid—only this was every day for two months without letup. I thought it would never end. And what little time there was when I didn't feel so sick, I was depressed and disoriented like I've never been before. Now that it's been months, I still feel scared, and my mind and body are both depleted. I know, in time, I'll get stronger. And when I'm finally able to see patients again, I'll certainly have a different attitude. It sure makes a difference seeing this kind of sickness from the other side of the bed!"

Getting Through Treatment: Emotional Survival Techniques

- *Find out everything you can—in advance.* Although this guideline could be taken to an extreme, it still pays to learn as much as possible about your treatment beforehand. This applies not only to hopeful information, such as cure rates, but also to threatening data, such as unpleasant side effects or pain during recovery. Research shows that patients who are well informed about side effects and pain have an easier time and use less pain medication than people who undergo the same treatment in a veil of ignorance. Knowing what is ahead helps you prepare emotionally.
- *Check out alternatives.* (This is a corollary of the first rule.) As you discover unpleasant side effects or complications of your treatment, particularly ones you especially fear, find out what you can *do* about them. For example, a young man undergoing chemotherapy for testicular cancer is likely to be sterile for about two years and may have reduced fertility thereafter. If he has plans for children, banking sperm in advance of treatment is a viable alternative. Likewise, men undergoing treatment for prostate cancer, which can cause erectile dysfunction, can investigate penile implants, vacuum pumps, and medications such as Viagra before surgery or radiation. Women facing removal of a breast can find out about combining mastectomy with reconstruction in one procedure, possibly helping them maintain a more favorable image of

their bodies. Again, knowing what lies ahead—and what you can do about it—aids in emotional preparation.

- *Let yourself be cared for.* When you are beset by serious illness, it is healthy and adaptive to allow others to attend to your needs. Don't try to do it all on your own.

- *Remember that psychotherapy and psychotropic medications are always available.* If depression or anxiety become overwhelming, ask for professional help. Both conditions are eminently treatable. And therapy can be flexible to meet your needs; for example, if you're too ill or tired to come to the psychiatrist's office, the phone works just fine.

- *Connect.* Hurting alone hurts worse than hurting with others. Support groups, whether in person, on the phone, or via e-mail, provide the opportunity to communicate with others in the same predicament. Being listened to—and listening—has a way of cutting anxiety down to size.

- *Pain is to be expected in cancer treatment, but suffering is unnecessary.* By *pain* I mean a tolerable level of discomfort; suffering refers to the kind of severe, agonizing, demoralizing hurt that tyrannizes you. Current medical technology makes suffering unnecessary with excellent medications for controlling pain and nausea. So don't be afraid to tell your physician or nurse how you feel and to ask for the medication you need.

- *Everyone can have some success with treatment.* Regardless of the severity of cancer, in this day and age, numerous treatment options exist. Perhaps one way of looking at cancer treatment is to view it as a mechanism to buy time until more effective, less toxic methods can be found. Cancer research is on an exceptional success curve. In the not too distant future, vaccines and gene therapy ("turning off" a malfunctioning gene) will be standard care.

6

SURVIVAL:
RETURNING TO "NORMAL"?

AS THE LEGEND GOES, Damocles was a courtier of Dionysius the Elder (431–367 B.C.), the autocratic ruler of the classical Greek colony of Syracuse on the island of Sicily. One day, Damocles made the mistake of telling Dionysius that rulers such as he had the best of all possible worlds: riches, power, and many servants at their beck and call. Dionysius, though, had a very different view of his life, and he didn't care for what he considered to be upstart impertinence. To teach Damocles a lesson in the reality of a ruler's lot, Dionysius invited Damocles to the place of honor at a banquet and set before him a marvelous meal. The guest enjoyed mightily all the many delicacies on his plate until he happened to look up. There above him hung a heavy battle sword, dangling by the hilt from a single, thin horsehair, its point aimed directly at him. Damocles was enjoying the delights of life—yet that same life could be snatched away in an instant's misfortune.

Anyone who has survived cancer knows exactly how Damocles felt. Survival brings the same delight Damocles felt upon seeing the sumptuous meal spread before him. After all, a serious disease has been surmounted, and life is again the survivor's to enjoy in all its many flavors. Yet over that joy hangs a dread made all the more keen by cancer's close encounter with mortality and the fear that the cancer may someday return.

This mix of feelings has a great deal to do with the power of survivorship. Throughout its course, cancer provides the opportunity to grow and stretch emotionally. Upon being freed from the rigors of treatment, one has the psychological, physical, and cognitive strength to reflect on priorities, relationships and health and to appreciate the beauty of the moment and the small pleasures of every day.

Shifting Gears as the Reality of Survivorship Takes Hold

Surprisingly, moving from treatment into survivorship can be as disturbing and stressful as facing up to diagnosis or choosing treatment. Often the transition comes suddenly. One day, you see your doctor, who lays a kind hand on your shoulder and says, "You're in remission. No reason to see you again for six months." And in that moment the world changes into something new. Suddenly you are again a "normal" person, someone who can enjoy doing everyday things. But, at the same time, a note of anxiety may creep into this new, deliciously normal way of life. For months, perhaps even years, your life has been defined by doctors' visits, laboratory tests, diagnostic and curative surgeries, chemotherapy infusions, and sessions under a radiation machine. You have lived in a strange network of physicians, nurses, social workers, medical assistants, and technicians. Now that world is gone, and you are on your own. Some people find themselves profoundly anxious at this separation from people they have come to know and depend on.

Although it can be difficult, you can make the change. A number of scientific studies of cancer survivors show that a large majority do very well, particularly after an adjustment period that lasts from months to two years after treatment. Typically people are able to pick up their lives where they left off, returning to their families, jobs, and social activities. But survivors face a number of physical and psychological issues. Like Damocles, they are feasting under a sword.

Survivorship includes a long list of potential physical problems. A common complaint is fatigue. The wear and tear on the body from surgery, chemotherapy, and radiation can produce a deep tiredness that lasts for several months to a year after treatment. A very small percentage of patients who have undergone extremely aggressive treatment report that their energy level never returns to what it was before they contracted cancer. Engaging in regular exercise and the judicious use of a stimulant such as Ritalin help make up for the loss.

Certain chemotherapy protocols, when used in very high doses, also may cause long-lasting, or, rarely, permanent nerve damage. The most common damage is neuropathy, which may cause tingling or pain in the extremities. Physical therapy and low doses of medication, such as the tricyclic antidepressant Elavil, are extremely useful for treating this problem.

Issues of fertility and sexuality are much more likely to become prominent in survivorship than they were during treatment. Treatment is so preoccupying that thinking about lovemaking or having another child merits low priority. In fact, having another child during this time may be prohibitive. That changes in survivorship, when the crisis of making it through treatment no longer gets in the way. However, loss of fertility—sometimes temporary and sometimes permanent—is a common complication of certain cancers and treatment. For example, sterility in women can result from radiation of the pelvis, a common therapy in the treatment of Hodgkin's disease. In men, treatment for testicular cancer may lead to transient or lifelong sterility.

Likewise, sexuality can change as a result of treatment. As we have seen, surgery for prostate or bladder cancer in men may result in erectile dysfunction or loss of the ability to ejaculate. Similarly, treatment for cervical or uterine cancer in women can change sexual response, making intercourse difficult or even painful.

This type of problem may be compounded in women whose ovaries are removed or who are treated with tamoxifen, which is often prescribed for women who have had breast cancer. These therapies can induce premature menopause, possibly leading to hot flashes, sweating, vaginal dryness, mood swings, and other symptoms of the change of life, often years before women had planned to deal with such issues.

The good news is that sexual issues can often be dealt with successfully. As we saw in the case of Ally and Michael in Chapter 5, sex therapy is effective at re-creating trust and openness and helping a couple find new ways to express intimacy. In the case of physically induced sexual difficulties, medications such as Viagra are excellent in treating erectile dysfunction in men, and lubricants such as Astroglide and Replense may reduce vaginal dryness in women.

Sometimes there are physical limitations. The loss of part or all of a limb may well mean that a favorite sport can no longer be played or that the simple act of getting up the stairs becomes an ordeal. There are a number of things you can do in addition to mourning the loss. One is to seek out a physical pursuit that bypasses the missing limb. For example, someone who has lost a lower leg can still swim, even if she or he can no longer jog. The key is to learn how to experience your body in new ways. Another strategy is to stay connected with the lost activity in a different manner, such as coaching a Little League team if you used to play baseball, or writing about an activity in which you once were actively involved. You can also pursue some long-desired pleasure you previously hadn't had time for, such as collecting old jazz albums or flower arranging. And there are certainly many examples of people who have overcome all obstacles and resumed the same vigorous physical activities in which they participated before the cancer.

There can be pain, usually as a result of surgery. A common example is chronic pain from abdominal surgery. Internal scar tissues called adhesions that can form following intestinal surgery may cause intermittent discomfort. Sometimes they can be repaired in follow-up surgery or by medication, but sometimes they are there to stay. People can learn to deal with chronic pain through mind-body techniques including formal programs created by Jon Kabat-Zinn and Herbert Benson (see Sources at back of book). Oncologists can refer patients to local programs.

Underlying all these realities of survivorship is a series of key psychological issues, some of which are unconscious—difficult to articulate yet powerful in their effects. And once they are understood, they can add to a survivor's ability to cope.

Feeling Bad About Feeling Good

Some cancer survivors find themselves feeling guilty over making it. They wonder why they have gone on living while others have died. This kind of response is most pronounced in people who are extremely empathic, take responsibility for others, are prone to guilt, or have experienced the death of loved ones from cancer.

A friend of mine who survived cancer—and who is now actually grateful to the disease for helping him reconsider his life priorities—described this survivor's guilt poignantly. "Two weeks ago," he said, "I attended a fund-raising dinner where the guest speaker was the child of a Jewish man who had lived through the Holocaust. The speaker said that her father was constantly tormented by guilt. 'Why,' he asked himself, 'had I survived, when the Nazis shot or gassed everyone else in my family?' He didn't have an answer. I had no trouble identifying with his dilemma. Especially when I am speaking to family members of people who have died after a bout of cancer, I feel almost embarrassed when the focus of the conversation turns to me and someone asks, 'So, what about you? How are *you* feeling?' Of course, I should say, 'I feel great!' because I do, but often there's this queasy feeling I associate with guilt. 'Why,' I ask myself, 'did I survive, when this person's wife or parent or child died?' The question troubles me, but I don't have an answer."

Truth is, nobody does. Often, even highly trained physicians have no idea why some people do poorly and die, whereas others with the same type of cancer do well and go on to full and productive lives after treatment. Rather than worry about the question, treat each day of your new life as an untouched canvas, and use it to paint your existence in deeper and richer colors.

Coming to Terms with a Different You

It is a universal aspect of the cancer experience that an individual comes out of treatment feeling different about his or her body. Obviously, this can be a realistic response: Someone who has lost a breast or lung to can-

cer surgery is certainly going to have a new body image. But this change
in self-perception also extends to cancers that cause few or no changes in
outward appearance. A research study found that more than one in four
persons who had survived Hodgkin's disease, a cancer that causes no long-
term change in appearance, felt they looked worse after cancer than
before. Similar results have been found in survivors of leukemia and bone
marrow transplant. It may be that these shifts in self-perception are connected to the loss in energy that often goes along with cancer survival.

Getting used to a new body image is particularly challenging when the
change cuts to the core of who you are. A striking example from my practice is Mary Ann, a divorced forty-year-old flight attendant who was
referred by her oncologist for evaluation of her anxiety. Diagnosed with an
aggressive breast cancer, Mary Ann had undergone a bilateral radical mastectomy about six months earlier, and had only recently completed a
course of chemotherapy. Mary Ann's hair was beginning to grow back, but
when I saw her for the first time she was still wearing a short blond wig
that was obviously not her own hair.

"I was doing just fine with this cancer thing until about a week after the
surgery," Mary Ann explained when I asked how she was doing. "Suddenly
I became frightened and nervous all the time. I jump at the slightest sound,
and the rest of the time I feel like I'm disconnected, walking around in a
daze. I can't sleep at night. Instead of dreaming, I have flashbacks of waking up in the recovery room right after my surgery. That was an awful
experience. I felt drugged and confused from the anesthetic, my chest
ached, and I knew there was less of me now than there had been. I keep
obsessing about the damage that's been done to my body, the mutilation.
Even my hair bothers me; I know it will grow back, but I keep touching
my head and, feel so self-conscious. Sometimes I feel like I'm going crazy."

Mary Ann wasn't going crazy. Rather, her feelings were a natural and
understandable response to the ordeal she had been through. Psychiatrists
call her emotional pattern *posttraumatic stress disorder,* a common syndrome
in cancer that we will discuss in more detail in Chapter 7. As Mary Ann and
I investigated her psychological history, some themes emerged over time to
explain why breast cancer treatment had been especially hard on her.

An only child with long blond hair and perfect features, Mary Ann was the apple of her father's eye. He even called her "my little beauty queen." During adolescence, Mary Ann turned into a dazzlingly pretty woman whose movie-star face and well-curved body drew constant attention from boys. Mary Ann enjoyed flirting; to her, it was fun. At the same time, though, she was becoming defined by her appearance, for while Mary Ann was an intelligent and good student, she thought of herself more in terms of beauty than brains. Intellect and personality had little to do with who she was; her face and her body created her identity. Family, boyfriends, and even the husband who eventually left her subtly reminded her that only her beauty made her valuable. Without it, they seemed to say, she was nothing.

Then came breast cancer. Mary Ann had lost not only her breasts and her hair; the core of her self-worth had been removed as well. She was cut down to the nothing she secretly always feared she would become if she ever lost her "beauty." Most of our sessions over several years in psychodynamic psychotherapy focused on redefining how Mary Ann had learned to value herself. Mary Ann came to see that she was more than her breasts and her hair. Her intelligence and warm personality moved to a central position in her self-perception. Slowly, she gained a balanced view of her emotional self. Her inner sense of self eventually led her to greater confidence, both personally and professionally. Although still aware of her appearance, Mary Ann had found a balance between external and internal attributes.

The body is an important determinant of self-image, but it is only one variable in a total positive sense of self. Over time, Mary Ann regained some of what she had lost. Her hair grew back, and her breasts were skillfully reconstructed with plastic surgery. Ironically, her cancer precipitated her acceptance of herself as a woman defined by goodness.

Engaging in a New Life

Even though the word *survivorship* is used as a possible synonym for *return to normal*, what does "normal" mean after cancer? After all, cancer *has* changed your life. But it also can present an opportunity for growth, if you look for it. People who have been through cancer often learn important lessons about the nature of life. But if they try to return to how they were *before* cancer, without identifying what they have learned and incorporating it into the way they live, they will find themselves in the midst of a difficult emotional crisis.

Dana was a good example. She never thought she would be sitting in a psychiatrist's office. But then again, she never thought she would have breast cancer.

Like Mary Ann, Dana was forty when she found out she had the disease. Until that moment, her life had seemed almost charmed. A mother of two, she was petite and athletic-looking, and was married to a caring man. Dana volunteered with Alzheimer's patients, a task she came to with great patience and generosity. As a practicing Jew and an active member of her synagogue, Dana found comfort and connection in her religion. Then, in the shower after an afternoon tennis match, Dana felt a small, hard lump in her right breast. Her world began to change.

Dana had a luckier time than Mary Ann. Her cancer was confined to a small area that could be taken out with a lumpectomy, and there was no evidence that the disease had spread into her lymphatic system. Following the surgery, Dana received chemotherapy for six months as added insurance. She tolerated the treatment very well, with only occasional nausea. Then she started taking tamoxifen and would continue to do so for several years. Although Dana disliked the menopause-like symptoms brought on by the drug, she was doing well physically.

Dana's doctor had pronounced her "cured," and her family and friends saw the same attractive, lively, and generous woman they had known before cancer. Dana knew she would have repeated follow-up examinations to detect any recurrence, but her physician had told her not to worry. The chance that the cancer might return was very small, according to the doctor. Dana agreed. She had taken on surgery and chemotherapy with the same determination, wit, and energy that she displayed throughout her life, and she had come out on the winning side. She thought little about cancer, and rarely did death cross her mind. Life until now had been good to her, so there was no reason to believe that it would be any less good in the future.

Yet something inside Dana had shifted. She tried to ignore the insidious signs of anxiety that started about two weeks after her last chemotherapy infusion. Then, on what seemed like an ordinary outing to the supermarket, Dana experienced her first panic attack. Out of the blue, her heart suddenly began to race, her breathing came fast and furious, her palms sweated, and she was consumed by the fear that she was about to die from a heart attack or stroke and by the desire to escape the market at all costs. Even though Dana avoided the supermarket after that, convincing her husband that he should do the shopping, the panic attacks continued—always unexpected, always profoundly disturbing. The anxious feelings accompanying these episodes and the worry about the next attack grew more intense and frequent, awakening Dana in the middle of the night and filling her with a strong sense of dread. When one of these attacks hit Dana while she was driving, forcing her to pull to the side of the road and leaving her bathed in sweat and fear, she knew she needed help. Her physician assured her that she was medically okay, then suggested that she might find a psychiatrist helpful. Thus, Dana came to me on the referral of her doctor, who accurately diagnosed her with panic disorder.

Dana took on our work together with the same energy she used to approach every challenge in her life. Quickly she came to see what was happening to her.

In a way, Dana's "easy" time with cancer left her draped in denial. Since she had suffered little psychologically or physically in the course of treatment, she was able to distance herself from cancer's emotional consequences. However, the psyche doesn't let us escape our emotional conflicts so easily. Dana's panic attacks following the conclusion of chemotherapy constituted what Sigmund Freud called *signal anxiety:* a message that the person contains a psychological imbalance. Just as the physical pain of a broken leg keeps us from walking on the damaged limb and doing it further harm, anxiety alerts us to an unhealthy psychological response.

As Dana started understanding what lay beneath her anxiety, her panic attacks began to ease. Before cancer, Dana had always felt in control of her life, but the disease had snatched that illusion away. Something foreign and potentially fatal had taken up residence inside her. Her body had moved outside the domain of her control—and so had her future. No matter how well Dana took care of herself, there was the small but nonetheless real chance that the cancer might come back.

This understanding stripped away Dana's denial of death. Like so many of us, she hadn't really believed that she was going to die someday. Cancer brought mortality home. And the anxiety she felt in response erupted as panic.

In psychotherapy, Dana did what we all must do if we are to live whole, full lives: She let herself understand that our existence has no certitude except for death itself, that control is myth, and that life is less owned than leased. Dana's world became more complicated, but ultimately she found it more intriguing, often poignant, and never boring. She found she had a greater capacity for engaging in all experiences—positive ones such as moments of joy with her family and negative ones such as sadness at the thought of cancer coming back.

The Fear of Recurrence—and the Resilience of the Human Spirit

Even if it fails to reach the high level of anxiety that prompted Dana's panic attacks, the fear that cancer can return underlies the psychological landscape for all survivors. They are reminded repeatedly of the reality that cancer recurrence may be detected every time they go in for a follow-up exam. Typically anxiety builds before the visit to the doctor and remains in the air until the test results come back. Then survivors can breathe a sigh of relief until the next follow-up exam. But a news story on cancer or a mention of the disease during a friendly conversation can trigger a powerful response of dread and anxiety. After all, anyone who has had the disease understands the anguish associated with it and has every reason to fear another episode.

In some people this dread takes the form that I call the "one-cell fear." The apprehension is that cancer treatment, no matter how thorough, has missed one malignant cell somewhere in the body. This single evil cell is looking for a place to attach and grow, and once it does, the disease will bloom again. The individual with one-cell fear lives in a state of anxious hypervigilance, frightened that the least sniffle, cough, or vague ache is the returning cancer's first sign. This fear can be carried to extreme lengths, usually for reasons that are more psychological than physical. An example of this is a forty-five-year-old man who had undergone a radical prostatectomy after a biopsy revealed early-stage cancer in his prostate. Fortunately, the pathology report found no cancer in the prostate or in the surrounding organs after surgery. Apparently, the multisite biopsy had removed all of the very small cancer. Even when the urologist informed the patient of these results and assured him that it was virtually impossible for the prostate cancer to return, the man walked about in a state of constant, low-level dread.

We all probably have cancer cells lurking in our bodies at this very moment. Fortunately, most of the time, our immune systems detect these cellular malignancies and eliminate them. Yet cancer survivors often take scant comfort in this reality and remain worried about the signs of possible disease, for cancer can return. And if anything can be worse than being told that you have cancer, it's being told that you have it again. Recurrence prompts a crisis of the same sort as diagnosis (see Chapter 4), with its initial numbness, followed by waves of depression, anxiety, and sleeplessness. The difference between initial diagnosis and early reactions to recurrence is that recurrence is often worse. Not only does it resurrect the old fears of pain, suffering, and death, but it brings back a cascade of memories from the initial cancer experience and destroys the optimism that accompanies survival. The result can be total demoralization.

But once the shock of recurrence passes, the survivor discovers that he or she has significant assets to draw on in this new round of disease. As a veteran of cancer treatment, the survivor knows how to prepare emotionally and physically for the experience. The logistics of treatment—setting and keeping appointments, preparing for surgery, getting to the infusion clinic, arranging child care, and the like—seem less overwhelming because they have been done before. More educated about the medical system, the survivor with recurrence is less likely to be buffaloed by bureaucracy and better equipped to get what he or she needs. And usually there is good news about treatment—more effective chemotherapeutic agents, perhaps a shift to hormone or immunotherapy, even a promising experimental treatment in a clinical trial.

In addition, survivors can shift their perspective on the disease. During the first encounter with cancer, most people say such things as "I'm going to beat this thing," because they see cancer as a discrete, single event to be overcome once and for all, something like a bout of pneumonia or a broken leg. In fact, cancer may be a chronic illness, a condition that comes and goes, not unlike some forms of arthritis. Care and treatment might be required for the remainder of life, and there will be good times as well as bad.

Recurrence often demonstrates the resilience of the human spirit. I have seen people experience repeated recurrences with chronic cancers, and each time they grow stronger. Although initially the emotions may be overwhelming, more often than not people use the crisis of recurrence as an opportunity for further maturation. They know what to do. The first thing is to return to the emotional antidotes that have worked in the past and discard the ones that haven't. Family and friends are important, and support groups, particularly with other people facing recurrence, can be very helpful. Finally, there is no place for guilt. Cancer can return, and *it's not the survivor's fault*.

Advice on Surviving Survivorship with Grace

- *Accept that you will be experiencing a range of emotional reactions.* Particularly early on in survivorship, you will be pulled in opposite directions. On the one hand, there is the fantastic sense of relief and the new freedom of "normalcy." On the other hand, there is concern over recurrence and, ironically, separation anxiety from the day-to-day medical system, mixed in with the paradox of the inevitable letdown that follows a battle fought well and won.
- *Know that a state of limbo lasts for a while.* The first few weeks or months of survivorship add up to an odd, disconcerting period when you are no longer an active cancer patient, yet not fully

returned to life. Don't judge what is happening or push it. Limbo will end in its own time.

- *Expect to be tired. Then expect your strength to return.* At first, don't demand too much of yourself or feel guilty that you can't immediately resume all responsibilities and activities. In time, though, you'll probably find that your stamina will return to normal as the full emotional import of survivorship makes its way into your psyche.
- *A million people will ask, "How are you feeling?"* The concern is touching, but unfortunately it comes right when you are trying to put distance between yourself and cancer. Don't take it personally.
- *And then they will forget to ask how you are doing.* After a while, people stop asking about your health. Again, don't take it personally, and don't let it hamper your growth.
- *Look back with family and friends.* Talk about both your experiences and theirs during diagnosis and treatment. All of you will have more emotional stamina for this discussion and a better perspective on it than you did during the actual crisis.
- *Take time to reflect.* If you objectively assess your efforts during diagnosis and treatment, you'll probably discover that you underestimated your coping skills beforehand and learned new ones in the course of dealing with the disease. This will give you new emotional strength and confidence.
- *Consult as needed.* If emotional symptoms trouble you, seek professional help. If your concerns focus on death, talk with members of the clergy. If you don't like organized religion, read or study philosophy instead. Just don't be afraid to seek help or guidance from other sources.
- *Relax.* Learn or continue to practice relaxation techniques such as yoga, the relaxation response, or meditation.
- *Play.* Have as good a time as you can at your level of energy. Start with the movies, then make it a short walk to notice nature, then try an afternoon stroll around the lake. Mount Everest can wait until next year.

When Death Is Inevitable: Journeying Toward Calm and Peace

As Dana discovered, we are all going to die. When cancer treatment fails to halt the disease, the reality of death hits home with suddenness and immediacy. How the patient responds depends on a number of factors.

Experience with the death of loved ones has much to do with the way one sees death. An individual who has watched his or her spouse die in agony from an advanced cancer is going to fear that the same fate awaits him or her. Likewise, someone who has witnessed only peaceful, calm deaths is less likely to experience fear.

Religious and spiritual beliefs are central. People of faith who have embraced the moral tenants of their belief system or who understand their passing as the pilgrimage to another world tend to be more peaceful and resigned than are those who see the end as only a cold void. Social and family connections are equally key. People who have given and taken nurturance from a circle of family and friends suffer less distress. Like anyone who is dying, they experience fear and grief at being separated from those they love, yet they are comforted by their intimate connections to loved ones and feel less alone.

When cancer becomes terminal, treatment shifts from curative to palliative: The goal is to keep the patient comfortable and functioning for as long as possible. As I have said earlier, pain is an inescapable part of daily existence, but suffering, either physical or psychological, is unnecessary. Good pain medication is available, and both psychotherapy and medication can be used to deal with the anxiety and depression that often arise in the late stages of disease.

As Elisabeth Kübler-Ross has explained in her marvelous, pioneering writings, people who are confronted with death and dying move through a number of mood states. Sometimes they are depressed, sometimes anxious, sometimes in denial, sometimes trying to bargain. Finally, most accept what is happening. In the final moments before death, all patients, no matter what their prior emotional state, make a remarkable transition into a state of complete calm. Not once have I seen a patient die scared. Rather, they are peaceful, serene, and composed.

I learned this from Mattie, the first dying patient whom I treated in psychotherapy. She was thirty, only two years older than I was at the time, then a senior resident in psychiatry. I met Mattie in the middle of the night, when she showed up at the ER. She was a small waif-like woman who had tried to kill herself with an overdose of pills. Suddenly frightened at the prospect of actually dying, she had a friend drive her to the hospital. I had to be awakened from a deep sleep to see her, and I was none-too-excited at the prospect.

"So," I asked, in a cool tone, "you want to tell me about this?"

"My boyfriend left me. He just up and took a hike. I couldn't stand it. So I took an overdose of Valium and aspirin."

As Mattie talked, I learned she was an urban planner who lived alone. She was obviously intelligent and quick-witted, and I was surprised that her boyfriend wanted out. I was more surprised that she wanted to die as a result.

"Why did you have the Valium?" I finally inquired, since it's a prescription medication often used for people with anxiety.

"My doctor prescribed it," Mattie said casually. "I was having some nervousness after I found out I have malignant melanoma."

I was shocked. "You have cancer?"

"I did. But I've had the surgery. So the chances of the cancer killing me are about the same as this ceiling falling."

I looked up at the warped, peeling tiles overhead and didn't feel totally reassured. "Maybe we should talk more about this," I suggested.

Over many months of psychotherapy sessions, Mattie revealed that she was indeed frightened that the cancer would recur and kill her. That fear and the depression it spawned, more than her emotional reaction to her boyfriend's departure, had precipitated her suicide attempt. She and I looked at the core beliefs that led to her predisposition for depression, and Mattie reevaluated who she was and what worth she brought to the world. She slowly came to see herself from the viewpoint of her many friends and relatives: as a warm, insightful woman with a terrific zest for life and a playful sense of humor. Over time, Mattie's self-respect deepened.

Then she and I learned something else: Her melanoma had metastasized to her brain. Mattie's condition was terminal, and she soon moved into the hospital to receive the palliative care she needed at the end of her life.

One morning, she came to my office after spending an overnight at a friend's apartment while out of the hospital on an evening pass. For a woman close to death, she was full of joy.

"What's up?" I asked. "You're in as good a mood as I can ever remember seeing you in."

"Well," she began, "I was at my friend's apartment, and we were sitting outside after dinner. I looked up at the stars and I started to cry. The sky was just so beautiful, and I was wondering how many more times I would see it. I realized I wasn't crying because I was depressed or lonely, but more because I would really miss living."

It amazed me that Mattie, who had once seemed so helpless, was now talking about her own death with calm and composure. She was ready to die as a woman who had embraced a newfound maturity.

"You know what was really funny?" she continued. "It seemed foolish to keep on crying when I realized I couldn't make out this beautiful sky through my tears. You know, you can't see the Big Dipper if you're crying." Mattie started to giggle, and her laughter drew me in. In seconds I was laughing too.

Mattie died not long afterward, in her sleep, comfortably, without pain. I missed her terribly. Together we had taken a brief journey that helped her live and die. It had helped me too, showing me once again how much the patient has to teach the doctor.

Moving Toward Mortality

The process of moving toward death is unique to each individual. While Mattie certainly died in her own unique way, there are some fundamental guidelines that can help anyone facing the terminal stage of cancer:

- *Feel all your feelings.* The famous death and dying researcher, Elisabeth Kübler-Ross, saw the movement toward the end of life as a series of discrete stages, such as denial, anger, bargaining, and acceptance. In fact, the steps are not that discrete, and the feelings run together, as Kübler-Ross would later acknowledge. The key to healing—that is, achieving a sense of personal wholeness in the face of mortality—is to let yourself experience *all* your emotions, both positive and negative.

- *Open yourself to the enormity of the experience.* Having cancer takes major effort. Give yourself credit for doing so much so well. Grieve over what you are losing. Feel pride in what you have done.
- *Review your life.* Allow yourself time to see where you have been and to take pleasure in all the things you have accomplished. Appreciate the truth that you have lived your life as well as you could have lived it.

Cancer's Good Fortune

For all its pain, anguish, and mortal reality, cancer actually has a positive side. The clinical experience of psycho-oncologists like myself and the scientific literature show that being treated for cancer has constructive psychological value. For example, one study found that almost three out of every four women who had had breast cancer reported that cancer had changed their lives for the better.

A common benefit is a shift in values and philosophy. Instead of seeing their lives as infinite, cancer survivors feel they have been given a second chance to examine priorities and explore areas of meaning and value. A workaholic corporate lawyer who always led his firm in billable hours gave up that distinction after a bout with cancer, devoting more of his time to his children. "I thought I had a balanced life before cancer, but it was all out of whack. Now I have things more in perspective," he said.

A second common benefit is a strengthening of religious and spiritual values. Many of the patients I have worked with have returned to childhood religious practices they had abandoned. A Jew who came back to his faith after a long talk with a rabbi working as a chaplain in the hospital where he was awaiting cancer surgery said, "It took cancer to make me see that I had walked away from something of great value. Cancer brought me back to my spiritual home."

Third, some survivors report that they feel more optimistic about the future, in part because the fear of death is less prominent and controlling. I remember a devoted mother who said she had always worried about which college her children would get into. "Now I know it doesn't really matter," she said. "They're good kids on their own. They'll do well wherever they go to school."

Finally, the good fortune of cancer is that it provides a unique possibility for emotional growth. Cancer is a wake-up call to view one's self, one's relationships, and the world from a more mature perspective and to live with greater intimacy and gratitude—for example, I recall a man wrapped in machismo and inhibition who caressed his wife's hands each time he underwent chemotherapy infusion. "I felt a tenderness toward her I'd never experienced before," he said. "I realized I wanted more of something that, before I had cancer, I didn't even know existed."

PART THREE

SPECIAL CONSIDERATIONS

7

The Emotional Disorders of Cancer and Their Treatment

CANCER POSES SUCH A MAJOR CHALLENGE to one's being, both physically and psychologically, that it is hardly surprising to find the disease associated with a variety of emotional disorders. In a sense, these conditions are further manifestations of cancer. And like those other manifestations, the emotional disorders that often accompany the disease can be treated very effectively. Psychiatrists and other mental health professionals have access to a wide variety of therapeutic techniques and medications that work well to alleviate the troubling symptoms of emotional disorders and allow an individual to heal and live much more normally.

But there is an important caveat to understand first: Emotional reactions to cancer occur across a continuum. Experiencing serious sadness and anxiety upon learning that one has cancer is usual and expected, and it does not add up to a disorder. The difference between that normal reaction and an emotional disorder such as major depression is largely a matter of how severe the emotional symptoms are, how long they last, and how profoundly they interfere with an individual's ability to function in family, social, work, or school situations.

This chapter describes the principal disorders that are likely to accompany cancer, beginning with the most common ones. Then it moves on to briefly describe the methods and techniques used to treat them, specifically psychotherapy and medication.

Adjustment Disorder

Adjustment disorder stands at a midpoint between normal coping, on the one hand, and a major emotional disorder, particularly depression and anxiety, on the other. It is something of a normal reaction that goes over the top.

Adjustment disorder always arises in reaction to a clear, identifiable stressor that occurred no more than three months before the onset of the symptoms. Cancer, of course, is just such a stressor. The individual reacts to the stressor in a way that creates noticeable distress in some basic activity, causing difficulty in work, family and personal relationships, hobbies, or the enjoyment of life, including sexuality. Usually adjustment disorder will resolve on its own within six months from the time the stressor ends or is removed. But if the stressor continues, as is the case with cancer, then the condition can last indefinitely.

The symptoms of adjustment disorder vary. Sometimes they tend toward depression and make themselves known as periods of sadness, teariness, feelings of hopelessness, and the like. They can also tend toward anxiety—nervousness, worry, rapid heart rate, or sweaty palms, for example. Often depressive and anxious symptoms are mixed, with the individual feeling not only nervous, but sleepless and sad, for example. A person's conduct, as well as his or her mood and emotions, may be disturbed. For example, a woman who usually loves to go shopping recreationally may find herself so immobilized by alternating sadness and anxiety that she cannot even imagine heading off to the mall.

Adjustment disorder is usually treated with psychotherapy. In some cases, medication is used as well.

Generalized Anxiety Disorder

Everyone experiences anxiety to one degree or another. It's the butterflies-in-the-stomach, cotton-in-the-mouth, sweat-in-the-palms feeling that arises when you feel sudden turbulence on an airplane, are about to open a letter to see if you passed the bar exam, or pick up the phone to call the oncologist about the latest test results. Anxiety serves a purpose over the short term: It mobilizes the body for sudden action at a time when danger or threat loom. But anxiety that hangs on and becomes both constant and chronic is a serious emotional problem.

Even under the best of circumstances, anxiety tends to peak at each stage of the cancer cycle. Studies of breast cancer patients, for example, show that anxiety increases when the tumor is found, peaks just before surgery, and continues at a high level immediately thereafter, then declines slowly over the first year of survivorship. This pattern appears to hold true regardless of whether the woman is undergoing a mastectomy or a lumpectomy, so apparently it is the fact of cancer more than the extent of surgery that prompts this anxiety.

The expected anxiety of the cancer cycle becomes a disorder requiring treatment when its symptoms become overwhelming. These symptoms fall into four areas:

1. *Apprehensive expectation:* Uncontrolled worry
2. *Motor tension:* Trembling, twitching, or feeling shaky; muscle tension, aches or soreness; restlessness; lack of stamina
3. *Autonomic nervous system hyperactivity:* Shortness of breath, increased heart rate, sweating or cold, clammy hands, dizziness, dry mouth, frequent urination, hot flashes or chills, trouble swallowing or a lump in the throat (globus hystericus).
4. *Vigilance:* Feeling keyed up, strong startle response, difficulty concentrating, trouble sleeping, irritability

What distinguishes generalized anxiety disorder from adjustment disorder with primarily anxious symptoms is its severity and duration. Simply, generalized anxiety disorder is worse and it lasts longer. As an example, consider Ben and Jeffrey, who were diagnosed with leukemia and undergoing bone marrow transplantation. Both men were the same age and had strong support from family and friends. During the outpatient stage of treatment, Ben became constantly worried, nervous, and jittery. At times these feelings were intense, but for the most part they were moderate and more distressing than immobilizing. Still, Ben felt too unstable to spend time with his friends—a clear sign that his emotional state was getting in the way of a normal life. He was diagnosed with adjustment disorder.

By contrast, Jeffrey found himself in a state of endless worry and apprehension, practically unable to sleep for more than a few minutes at a time, extremely irritable, and so fearful that a car backfire triggered a potent startle response out of him. Jeffrey had experienced prior bouts of severe anxiety, and his symptoms were so distressing that he cut off all social contact, stayed home for days on end, and missed doctor's appointments because he was too anxious to leave the house. Jeffrey was diagnosed with generalized anxiety disorder.

Anxiety responds well to psychotherapy, which is often combined with medication. Relaxation techniques, such as the ones discussed in Chapter 2 as coping mechanisms, are effective as an adjunct treatment.

Major Depression

Depression is something like the blues to the extreme. While everyone hits low points that usually last only a few days, major depression is a bottomless pit that goes on and on. It is an abnormal, persistent mood state characterized by sadness, melancholy, slowed mental processes, and changes in such physical patterns as eating and sleeping. While feelings of being blue or down usually improve on their own after a few days, these feelings are ever-present in major depression.

Medically, depression is defined as the daily presence for two weeks of at least five of the following nine symptoms. One of the symptoms must be either melancholy mood or loss of pleasure in activities:

1. Melancholy mood or sadness (sometimes experienced as apathy or irritability for most of the day)
2. Loss of pleasure in practically all activities, particularly ones the person previously enjoyed (referred to as *anhedonia*)
3. Disturbed appetite, or either weight gain or loss
4. Disturbed sleep, particularly an inability to sleep through the night (insomnia)

5. Slowed or agitated physical activity
6. Fatigue or very low energy, often leading to a diminished or nonexistent sex drive
7. Feelings of worthlessness, low self-esteem, or guilt
8. Difficulty concentrating and thinking
9. Morbid or suicidal thoughts or actions

Rarely, in very severe cases, depressed people may develop psychotic symptoms. These can include false perceptions (hallucinations), such as hearing voices that tell them to hurt themselves, and false beliefs (delusions), such as believing that they deserve to be harmed.

The difference between adjustment disorder with depressive symptoms and major depression is, as with anxiety, a matter of degree and duration. In adjustment disorder, symptoms are likely to be a mood of continuing sadness that makes one less interested in social contacts and interferes with work or school. Depression is more of the same, only worse. The sadness is severe, sleeping difficulty is usually pronounced, weight is lost or gained suddenly, and the impairment of functioning may be so profound that the individual can hardly work or take part in ordinary daily activities. Some people are so immobilized by depression that they literally cannot get out of bed in the morning. The more severe the depression, the more likely are suicidal thoughts. Plans to harm oneself are *not* a sign of terminal cancer. Rather, they signal severe depression, even in people who are in the late stages of disease.

Depression is remarkably treatable. Psychotherapy, medication, or a combination of the two are used.

Posttraumatic Stress Disorder

Mary Ann, the flight attendant we talked about in Chapter 6 who had lost both breasts to cancer and kept experiencing flashbacks to her postsurgical experience in the recovery room, exhibited a classic case of posttraumatic stress disorder (PTSD). PTSD most recently entered the general vocabulary after returning combat veterans from the Vietnam War found themselves incapable of coping with daily life and often experienced battlefield flashbacks so vivid that they thought they had returned to the fighting in Southeast Asia. PTSD in people with cancer is the same disorder, with the disease substituting for the incoming fire of combat. In each case, a trauma that threatens death or serious injury occasions a series of specific symptoms. Typically, the disorder begins within three months of the trauma, but onset may be delayed for six months or longer. Its severity and duration vary. The disorder is considered acute if symptoms have been present for three months or less, and chronic if they have existed for more than three months.

The most prominent sign of PTSD is the reexperiencing of the traumatic event. Thoughts are intrusive, recurring, and distressing. They can come in a number of forms: disquieting flashbacks (vivid recollections of the trauma), amnesia (in which the person forgets where he or she is), nightmares, or powerful emotional reactions to small cues associated with the trauma, such as news reports on cancer or the smell of disinfectant in a physician's office. Because the thoughts and flashbacks associated with the trauma are so unpleasant, the individual with PTSD tries to avoid any person or situation connected with the event. The individual experiences a numbing of feelings, which may lead him or her to block out certain aspects of the memory of the trauma, feel uninterested in pleasurable activities, and avoid social contact. Finally, a person with PTSD is highly aroused and vigilant. Sleep is difficult, concentration is often impossible, and anger or irritability is constant. The normal startle response is highly exaggerated and extreme.

Treatment of PTSD consists of psychotherapy to increase awareness of the underlying emotions and beliefs and often medication to alleviate the symptoms. The disorder is quite common among cancer patients, although it is often overlooked. If the condition is recognized promptly, the outlook for treatment is very good.

Aaron, a twenty-eight-year-old chef, is a good example. When his surgeon called me, both puzzled and concerned, it had been six weeks since she had operated on Aaron to excise an abdominal tumor. The surgeon was most pleased with the outcome: The tumor was localized and the malignancy was only low-grade. Aaron had an excellent prognosis and required no further treatment. But he continually complained of insomnia, which, according to the surgeon, didn't respond to the sleep medications she had prescribed.

I saw Aaron the day after speaking with his surgeon. When I said hello and shook his hand in the waiting room, he fit the classic image of someone in the physiologic overdrive of fight-or-flight. Aaron was tense, restless, and sweaty. His dilated pupils scanned both me and the room.

When we began to talk in my office, Aaron was able to describe his current state articulately, although he was still tense. He said, "I haven't been the same since the surgery." With a little prompting from me, he said that significant anxiety had begun within days of the operation. His thoughts were filled with vivid, persistent recollections of being wheeled into the operating room and of lying in the recovery room confused, nauseated, and unable to speak because he was still intubated. Over the ensuing weeks, his days were full of poorly controlled pain, his nights with recurring nightmares of surgery and the recovery room.

"It wasn't that I couldn't sleep," Aaron said. "It was that I was too damn scared of those nightmares to *go* to sleep! And I felt so ashamed and confused that I couldn't bring myself to tell my surgeon that I never took the sleeping pills."

Aaron seemed somewhat relieved to get his story out. That gave me the opportunity to educate him about PTSD and reassure him that the disorder is both common and highly treatable. Learning that relieved some of his anxiety immediately.

Aaron underwent several sessions of supportive psychotherapy that gave him an opportunity for catharsis (basically, an opportunity to talk so as to get the trauma off of his chest), and he learned techniques for progressive muscle relaxation and breathing exercises to combat anxiety. In addition, I referred him to a postoperative support group at the hospital so that he could realize he was not alone in his frightened reaction to cancer surgery.

Panic Disorder

You may recall from Chapter 6 the story of Dana, a breast cancer survivor who found herself so overtaken by seemingly unexplained, severe anxiety that she had to pull over to the side of the road. She was experiencing a panic attack, the hallmark of panic disorder. There are fourteen possible symptoms of a panic attack, of which four or more must be present:

1. Sudden extreme nervousness that seems to come out of the blue
2. Palpitations, pounding heart, or accelerated heartbeat (*tachycardia*)
3. Sweating
4. Trembling or shaking
5. Feeling short of breath or smothered
6. Feelings of choking
7. Pain or discomfort in the chest
8. Distress in the abdomen or nausea
9. Feeling dizzy, light-headed, faint, or unsteady
10. A sense of unreality, as if events are happening in a movie or dream, or depersonalization, as if they are happening to someone else
11. Fear of losing control or going crazy
12. Fear of dying, typically by heart attack or stroke
13. Numb or tingling hands or feet
14. Chills or hot flashes

Panic attacks come on very suddenly, peak within seconds to minutes, then fade. Usually the whole experience lasts no more than ten or fifteen minutes.

The experience of one panic attack is not enough to support a diagnosis of panic disorder. Attacks have to be repeated and recurring, although no precise number in a given period of time has yet been specified. It matters, too, how the individual reacts to panic attacks. In true panic disorder, at least one attack prompts worry about subsequent attacks for a month or more. In addition, the individual with panic disorder reshapes his or her life to avoid situations where panic attacks seem more likely. In many individuals this develops into *agoraphobia,* a fear of public, open spaces such as schools, shopping malls, and sports stadiums.

Although unpleasant, a single panic attack is not dangerous. However, repeated, untreated panic attacks may increase the risk of cardiovascular disease, such as high blood pressure (*hypertension*) or abnormal heart rate and rhythm *(arrhythmia)*. Treatment usually consists of psychotherapy often combined with medication, and it provides excellent outcomes.

Phobia

Essentially, a phobia is a persistent, irrational, and exaggerated fear. The fright is so powerful that it causes immense distress to the individual, who will often go to great lengths to avoid the feared object or situation. In life outside cancer, phobias may attach to snakes, spiders, knives, and the like; in cancer, they arise around aspects of diagnosis or treatment. Conditioned nausea or vomiting in anticipation of a chemotherapy session is a classic case of phobia.

Phobia can be treated very effectively. Behavioral techniques, such as desensitization, are commonly used. In this approach, the person is introduced to the feared stimulus, such as the sight or smell of the infusion clinic, step by step, and is taught to relax as anxiety builds. Repeating the process over and over gradually robs the stimulus of its feared quality and reduces overall anxiety. Relaxation techniques are also useful, as is hypnosis by a trained professional. In the relaxed, suggestible state of hypnosis, the patient can be led to imagine the feared situation and can be taught how to relax as anxiety rises. This type of hypnosis is safe and effective and will not lead the patient to do anything against his or her will.

Delirium

I have mentioned delirium before—the state of confusion and disorientation that sometimes results from medical or surgical treatment for cancer as well as from the disease itself. Whereas adjustment disorder, major depression, generalized anxiety disorder, PTSD, panic disorder, and phobia are often *emotional* responses to cancer as a stressor, delirium is a *physical* reaction to the disease or its treatment.

Delirium has a number of symptoms. The hallmarks are confusion, disorientation, and the inability to sustain attention. Typically the person is restless, anxious, and irritable, and has trouble sleeping. The condition develops quickly and fluctuates rapidly, for example, worsening as the day progresses. The individual may be either highly active or extremely lethargic, and his or her emotional state is fast-changing, frightened, sad, angry, or euphoric. Delusions and hallucinations are common, and thinking and speech are disorganized and at times incoherent. Often the person cannot remember anything new.

Delirium in cancer has a number of possible causes. A cancerous tumor of the brain can cause the condition, as can organ failure or a change in electrolytes, such as calcium or sodium. An infection resulting in high fever is another possibility. And delirium can result as a side effect from certain chemotherapy agents, radiation of the brain, painkilling medications, and anesthetics.

Practically all deliriums are rapidly reversible. Treatment consists of helping the individual reorient to his or her surroundings and administering medications that counteract the confusion and disorientation. With treatment, delirium usually lasts no more than a week, although it may take up to a month for all cognitive functions to return to normal.

Organic Mood Disorder

Like delirium, an organic mood disorder results from physical changes rather than an emotional or psychological response to disease. Usually, overall mood shifts to depression, but sometimes the shift is manic—that is, highly energized and euphoric.

Organic mood disorder can have a number of causes. Some of the medications used in cancer treatment can be the cause, including opiates (used for pain control), propranolol (for high blood pressure and migraines), and steroids (for anti-inflammatory and anticancer properties). Also, a number of chemotherapeutic agents can be the culprit. They include interferon (used for malignant melanoma), procarbazine (for various cancers), tamoxifen (for breast cancer), and vincristine (for various cancers).

Another cause is either overactivity of the thyroid gland—which may produce excitement, or even mania—or underactivity—which can lead to lethargy and depression. Uncontrolled pain, anemia, and various metabolic imbalances also can induce organic mood disorder.

The difficult part of organic mood disorder is distinguishing it from depression or anxiety, which are more rooted in psychological causes. The difficulty is that symptoms are the same. The key to accurate diagnosis is checking through the physical causes to see whether any of them apply to the particular patient.

One patient I treated was Ann, an upbeat and optimistic young woman who was undergoing aggressive treatment for malignant melanoma, which included the immunotherapy agent, interferon. By disposition, Ann was a strong-willed woman with an athlete's fighting spirit, so it surprised everyone around her when she gradually became depressed as each new cycle of treatment began. Her mood shifted from energized to listless and flat; she had no interest in friends, and slept up to fourteen hours a day. It was clear to me that Ann's depression had little to do with her emotional history and everything to do with the interferon. A course of antidepressant medication resolved the problem promptly, lifting Ann's mood and allowing her to enjoy her life even during treatment.

Another patient, Maurice, underwent a mood swing in the opposite direction. His mood was understandably low and angry when he was first diagnosed with multiple myeloma, a cancer of the immune system's plasma cells. By the time he entered treatment, however, he was focused and resolved. However, one of the medications in his chemotherapy protocol was prednisone, a powerful steroid that is similar in its action to hormones secreted by the adrenal gland. After each treatment, Maurice became strikingly irritable and anxious and was beset by troubling heart palpitations, sweaty palms, and stomach butterflies. Both Maurice's oncologist and I suspected that the problem was the prednisone. To counteract its effects, an antianxiety medication was prescribed, which Maurice took only for several days following each chemotherapy treatment. This approach, coupled with reassurances to Maurice that he wasn't at fault for his emotional condition, improved matters greatly.

Organic mood disorder is treated by eliminating or changing any medication that is causing the problem, administering an antidote if necessary, and treating the underlying metabolic condition.

Mild Neurocognitive Disorder

Yet another disorder with a physical or biological basis, cognitive disorder affects the thinking aspects of mental function. Mild neurocognitive disorder requires that at least two of the following conditions hold true for at least two weeks:

1. Impaired memory, evidenced by a reduced ability to learn or to recall information
2. Disturbance in planning, organizing, sequencing, abstracting, and other so-called executive functions of the mind
3. Poor attention or greatly lowered speed in information processing
4. Impaired perceptual-motor abilities, such as difficulty in coordinating eye and hand movements
5. Decreased language ability, such as poor comprehension or elementary word choice

Mild neurocognitive disorder primarily has the same causes as delirium: a cancerous tumor of the brain, organ failure, an infection resulting in high fever, certain chemotherapy agents, radiation of the brain, painkilling medications, or anesthetics. Treatment consists of finding the underlying cause and addressing it. If the disorder is permanent, which happens rarely, cognitive retraining techniques, such as those used in head trauma centers, are effective at improving the patient's condition.

Substance Abuse

The emotional stress of cancer, possibly combined with a prior history or inborn predisposition to use drugs addictively, can lead to abuse at any point during the cancer cycle. Various drugs may be used, including alcohol, marijuana, narcotics, sleep aids, and antianxiety medications. Often an insidious problem that is hard to recognize, substance abuse can begin innocently, for example, in those taking much-needed pain medication.

Cancer caught Patrick when he had no time. Only thirty years old and already the president of a fast-growing dot-com company, Patrick worked endless hours and enjoyed the life of a single man in his limited spare time. Chronic headaches, which at first he attributed to overwork and too many late-night glasses of wine, forced him to see a doctor. Several weeks and seemingly dozens of tests later, Patrick was diagnosed with a brain tumor. He underwent both surgery and radiation, which left him emotionally empty and profoundly unhappy. He also was suffering a good deal of pain, for which he was prescribed Percodan, a powerful narcotic analgesic. The medication controlled the pain and took the edge off Patrick's despair, at times even inducing mild euphoria. He also liked the mood effect. Without telling his doctors what he was doing, Patrick began taking higher and higher doses, which left him not high but numb. He also used the pills to forestall the anxiety, flu-like symptoms, and cravings that narcotic withdrawal brought on. Patrick had become addicted.

As many substance abusers do, Patrick became good at manipulating his doctors. He obtained multiple prescriptions from his internist, surgeon, and radiation oncologist, none of whom checked with one another and all of whom saw only a responsible man in pain.

The situation continued until one of Patrick's friends, who was a recovering alcoholic, noticed five medication containers lined up on his coffee table. The friend respectfully confronted Patrick, who denied any problem. The friend didn't let go. He spoke to Patrick's family, and together they were able to persuade him to look at what was happening. Finally, Patrick joined Narcotics Anonymous, where he learned how to give up his drug habit. Ironically, he found out he no longer needed the medication for pain. Ordinary ibuprofen and relaxation exercises proved sufficient to control the discomfort that still bothered him periodically.

Only a small minority of the cancer patients who use analgesics or other psychotropics become addicted. Still, the problem can arise, particularly where this is prior use or a family history of addiction. Also, people who are impulsive or excessive risk takers and who lack effective coping skills are at risk.

Underlying Disorders

Psychological life doesn't start over when cancer is diagnosed. Indeed, the disease can exacerbate any emotional disorder already present in the individual's history, even if that disorder had been well controlled previously. People who have been depressed are more likely to get depressed again, for example, and those with a history of obsessive-compulsive disorder might find themselves developing intrusive, anxiety-provoking, repetitive thoughts and behavior. Fortunately, the problems respond well to treatment; since there is a prior history, a previously effective treatment plan may be implemented quickly.

Obsessive-Compulsive Disorder (OCD), although it rarely develops during cancer, can sometimes be a factor if it has been a previously underlying condition. *Obsessions* are recurrent and persistent thoughts and images that are experienced by the individual as intrusive and inappropriate and cause marked anxiety (e.g., thinking about whether he/she turned off the coffee pot at work, keeping him/her awake each night for hours at a time). *Compulsions* are repetitive behaviors (e.g., hand washing) or re-checking, (e.g., checking a door lock over and over) which an individual feels he/she cannot control. The individual realizes that both behaviors are excessive and unreasonable but simply can't control them. Refer back to Deborah's case, in Chapter 4, for an example.

The Talking Treatment: Psychotherapy

In one or another of its many forms, psychotherapy has a role in the treatment of most cancer-related emotional disorders. The word *psychotherapy* comes from two Greek roots meaning "treat the mind," and that's precisely what psychotherapy aims to do. Psychological techniques are used to resolve symptoms and treat the underlying causes of emotional disorder.

Sometimes psychotherapy is called talk therapy, to set it apart from the use of medication alone. Talking plays a role in psychotherapy: Typically the patient discusses symptoms, concerns, and feelings with the psychotherapist, who listens carefully and provides feedback and insight.

Two aspects of psychotherapy distinguish it from other types of helping relationships, such as career or academic counseling. One is the *therapeutic alliance,* which refers to the agreement between the patient and the psychotherapist to work together toward a goal. This agreement allows the psychotherapist to offer specific suggestions and insights, and it gives the patient the space to listen even if the ideas raise negative or hostile feelings. The therapeutic alliance removes the usual barriers to understanding the self and permits change at a deep emotional level.

The second aspect is *transference.* As therapy proceeds, the patient's prior repressed feelings about significant figures in his or her past—such as anger or warmth toward a parent, or love or jealousy toward a sibling—shift unconsciously onto the therapist. The patient actually begins to deal with the therapist as if he or she were the parent or sibling. The psychotherapist, however, doesn't behave as the parent or sibling once did. Rather, he or she can reflect back the feelings to the patient as a way of demonstrating what is happening emotionally. Transference both reveals previously hidden feelings and reactions and helps the patient find new ways of dealing with them.

Psychotherapy in its modern form has been around for a little over a century, dating to the work of an Austrian physician, Josef Breuer, who later collaborated with and influenced Sigmund Freud (1856–1939), the father of classical psychoanalysis. Freud's studies and writings laid the foundation for modern psychotherapy. Practically every contemporary psychotherapeutic technique derives from his approach.

What happens in psychotherapy depends largely on the training of the individual psychotherapist and the type of therapy he or she is using.

Psychodynamic Psychotherapy

Rooted in Freud's ideas that current emotional issues originate in the unresolved, unconscious conflicts of early life, psychodynamic psychotherapy focuses on exposing unconscious feelings from childhood through transference and other techniques. Patient and therapist sit facing each other (unlike classical psychoanalysis, in which the patient lies on a couch and the therapist sits out of the patient's view) to allow direct interaction between them.

Another form of this technique is called brief psychodynamic psychotherapy, which is less time-consuming because it focuses on specific goals and outcomes rather than a comprehensive elucidation of the patient's psyche. Brief psychodynamic psychotherapy can be very effective in treating adjustment disorder, major depression, and generalized anxiety disorder rooted in the individual's psychological history.

Cognitive-Behavioral Therapy

Cognitive-behavioral therapy (CBT) melds the insights and techniques of two closely related schools of psychology. Behavioral therapy began in the 1950s, largely as a result of the work of psychologist B. F. Skinner, Ph.D. According to Skinner, all emotional disorders are learned responses to feared stimuli. Cognitive therapy originated in the 1960s in the depression research of Aaron Beck, M.D. Freud believed that how we feel determines how we think, but Beck reversed this formulation, maintaining that thinking determines feeling—that is, what we believe about ourselves and how we obtain information about the world, determine our emotional state. These premises about self and surroundings, which are every bit as unconscious as long-repressed childhood emotions, are the determinants of feeling.

Instead of journeying back into the emotions of childhood, cognitive-behavioral therapists emphasize the here and now. Therapy sessions focus on uncovering the negative thought patterns (cognitive distortions) that underlie emotions. As these come out, the patient is given homework (typically, exercises to identify and explore the validity of the hidden unrealistic cognitions and to recognize them for what they are). Relaxation training is often used to help deal with fears connected to these beliefs.

Cognitive-behavioral therapy can be very effective against depression, anxiety, panic disorder, and adjustment disorder. It has the advantage of working quickly and being a good adjunct to medication.

Behavior therapy, by itself, utilizes learning theory to remove symptoms through the use of reconditioning techniques. It is particularly helpful for phobias and anticipatory nausea prior to chemotherapy treatment.

Interpersonal Therapy

Pioneered by Gerald Klerman, M.D., and John Markowitz, M.D., of the Weill Medical College of Cornell University, interpersonal therapy (IPT) emphasizes the importance of current and past relationships in emotional disorders. Developed originally as a research tool, this therapeutic approach examines the conflicts, distortions, and difficulties in current relationships with other people and with one's environment. The crux of IPT is the link between mood and life events. Interpersonal therapy works toward the goals of increased self-esteem, decreased symptoms, and enhanced social function.

IPT can be useful in treating the depression and anxiety in cancer patients that arises from feeling as if their lives are out of control. With cancer, IPT focuses mainly on *role transition,* helping the patient accept the loss of an old, familiar role (being physically well) and the beginning of a new, still-unknown role (being a patient). This perspective helps the patient understand and more readily manage the apparent chaos of change.

Supportive Therapy

The form of therapy that is the most like career or academic counseling, supportive therapy provides the patient with advice, guidance, and direction about the here and now. Basically the therapist says, "Here's what's happening. Let's discuss what you can do about it." Supportive therapy bolsters the individual's healthy defense mechanisms as tried and true ways of coping with stress. For example, if denial or intellectualization is working, it is reinforced.

Supportive psychotherapy is often useful for the individual who would not seek out psychotherapy if it were not for the stress of cancer. This approach requires less belief in the laws of psychology than other forms of talk therapy, and is not threatening to those who seek symptom relief without probing.

Psychoeducation

A related technique, psychoeducation aims to reduce symptoms by clearing up misinformation and misperceptions about emotional disorders. The therapy provides emotional support, the chance to express feelings in a safe setting, and the opportunity to gain mastery and control through learning more about the emotional disorders. Even less threatening than supportive therapy, psychoeducation is almost like taking a college course. The didactic approach provides cancer patients with important information about the emotional consequences of their medical condition, including how to identify warning signs and respond to a crisis. It also educates family members who attend the sessions.

Group Therapy

Group therapy does just what the name implies. Instead of a single person meeting one-on-one with a therapist, people with similar concerns meet with a therapist or therapists and discuss their common issues. Many therapists like group therapy because, at times, it reaches more people faster. Patients benefit because they draw not only on the expertise of the therapist but also on the insights and experiences of the other participants. By building strong bonds among the participants, group therapy helps eliminate the social isolation that can accompany cancer. Research by David Spiegel, M.D., and his colleagues at Stanford showed that group therapy for terminally ill breast cancer patients helped women live longer and better.

Family Therapy

Focusing not so much on the individual patient as on the family system in which the patient lives, family therapy can be a very powerful and effective technique. The therapist involves the entire family in the process, focusing on the roles each person plays in both adaptive and maladaptive patterns. It is a good approach for medical crises affecting the family (for example, when a patient returns home after extensive and disabling surgery), circumstances where family support for the patient is problematic, or situations where another family member experiences a psychological crisis because of the cancer (such as a young child becoming disruptive in school as a result of his father's prostate cancer).

Brief Crisis Counseling

This type of therapy focuses on dealing with the immediate problems presented by one of cancer's many crises—diagnosis, for example, or making a tough therapeutic choice about whether to undergo a stem cell transplant. Often such a crisis can precipitate adjustment disorder. The focused approach of brief crisis counseling is an excellent way of dealing with such symptoms as sleeplessness, anxiety, and sad mood brought on by the crisis. The therapist's goal is to restore the individual to the level of functioning he or she enjoyed before the crisis, often with guidance for distress arising from pain, uncertainty about prognosis, and changes in relationships. Like supportive psychotherapy, brief crisis counseling relies on the individual's own constructive defense mechanisms as tried-and-true ways of handling stress.

Marital and Sex Therapy

Cancer places a weighty burden on even the most perfect marriage and has a way of exposing the cracks in all the rest. Marital therapy, also known as couples counseling or marriage counseling, focuses on the relationship between the two lovers, both of whom meet with the psychotherapist. Research has shown that couples therapy is more effective at resolving the communications issues common in marital problems than is individual therapy for one or both partners.

Sex therapy may be used in conjunction with marital therapy for couples with sexual complaints, or it may be used alone. Various cancer treatments can disrupt or change a couple's sexual patterns, either because of shifts in body image or changes in the sexual organs due to surgery, medication, or radiation. The goals of sex therapy are to help the couple relearn each other's bodies and to develop new ways of touching and communicating. Typically the therapist gives the couple homework assignments. In the privacy of their home, they engage in nonsexual body exploration. Then, as trust develops and communication improves, the interaction becomes increasingly sexual. Sex therapy can be strikingly effective at overcoming fears about sexual performance and behavior, particularly during survivorship.

Talking Can Help

The bottom line on psychotherapy is reassuring. Given the number of available effective techniques, there is an effective way to treat practically all the psychological symptoms that arise in cancer. In addition, psychotherapy offers patients who are interested the opportunity to explore their own psyches more deeply. Cancer holds the paradoxical promise of deepening one's life—and psychotherapy can help deliver on that promise.

Medicines for the Mind

Over the past fifty years, psychiatrists have become increasingly successful at treating major emotional disorders, in large measure because of medications that have become available. Medicines for the mind— or, technically, psychotropic drugs—are sometimes used alone, but commonly they are combined with psychotherapy. Psychotherapy and medication together are often more effective than either modality on its own.

The number of medications is so extensive that providing a detailed rundown would fill a book at least as large as this one. This chapter gives an overview of the basic types of psychotropic medications and their uses. This treatment in cancer patients may be complicated. Yet, in the hands of a skilled physician, such medicines can be of utmost help in providing emotional comfort.

Antidepressants

Prozac made antidepressants a household word, but there are more medications in this group than that one famous brand name. Antidepressants are, as the name states, medications that counteract depression. They also work well against panic disorder and posttraumatic stress disorder.

Prozac is a selective serotonin reuptake inhibitor (SSRI). It works at the level of the brain cell, slowing the rate at which the cell utilizes the chemical messenger (neurotransmitter) serotonin and allowing the serotonin level to increase. The effect of that buildup is a decrease in the symptoms of depression, although SSRIs take one to four weeks to work once an adequate dose has been reached. They generally have fewer side effects than some of the other antidepressants, but they can make some people feel anxious or sedated, cause an upset stomach, and lessen libido. SSRIs are generally safer, even if taken in overdose, than other antidepressants.

Tricyclic antidepressants (TCAs) also affect the activity of serotonin and another neurotransmitter known as norepinephrine. They are very useful against depression and are also indicated for panic disorder. In addition, they have pain-reduction properties, which increases their usefulness in cancer treatment. Side effects can be a problem, as TCAs may dry out the mouth, cause constipation, blur vision, cause urinary difficulties and sexual dysfunction, and lead to weight gain. Fortunately, antidotes exist for the side effects of all psychotropics.

Monoamine oxidase inhibitors (MAOIs), the first of the antidepressants to be developed, increase brain levels of serotonin, norepinephrine, and perhaps dopamine. They are usually used in patients who cannot tolerate or respond to other antidepressants. Side effects include change in sexual responsiveness, weight gain, and postural hypotension—a feeling of light-headedness or dizziness upon standing up. Although very useful, the biggest problem with MAOIs is that they can cause a sudden, potentially life-threatening increase in blood pressure when combined with certain foods and drugs: People on MAOIs have to avoid ripened cheeses, aged meats, and wine because they contain a chemical (tyramine) that can interact with the MAOI and boost blood pressure. Medications that raise blood pressure, such as over-the-counter decongestants, have to be avoided, and MAOIs can also interact with some of the medications commonly used in cancer treatment. As a result, they are rarely prescribed for people who have complex medical disorders.

Another group of antidepressants include the novel, or heterocyclic, antidepressants—so named because of their chemical structure—which are hybrids of SSRIs and TCAs. They provide useful alternative treatment options.

Finally, stimulants such as Ritalin and Dexadrine, although not widely prescribed or particularly useful for depression in the general population, work remarkably well for the medically ill. They have a rapid effect, which may make them a better choice than the slower-onset antidepressants. They need not be used for long time periods, and, contrary to popular belief, they are rarely addictive.

Neuroleptics

Neuroleptic medications, which are also called major tranquilizers, are commonly used to treat schizophrenia and psychotic depression. They are extremely effective in ameliorating symptoms of delirium in cancer patients. There are two groups: the original medications, known as typicals, and the newer group, named novels or atypicals, because they have a different mechanism of action. Neuroleptic medications are extremely potent drugs with many side effects, particularly Parkinson-like problems including stiffness, slowed motor movements (for example, difficulty walking), tremors, and restlessness. Although the novel neuroleptics have fewer side effects, all should be used for the shortest possible time period.

Antianxiety Medications

Again, the name describes the function. These medications are also known as minor tranquilizers or anxiolytics, which means "anxiety dissolvers." Most of the anxiolytics commonly used in cancer-associated disorders are benzodiazepines, a large family of medications that include such well-known brand names as Valium and Xanax. Long used as psychotropic medications, benzodiazepines are quick-acting and effective, but they may leave the patient feeling drugged or sedated. Usually this effect moderates within several days as the body adjusts to the medication. Benzodiazepines may decrease libido, and they interact with alcohol, so drinking must be restricted or avoided. They also pose a potential risk of addiction and withdrawal, so they should not be used over the long term if possible. Additionally, most anxiolytics are usually effective as sleeping aids. Two nonbenzodiazepines are also available: Buspar is a nonsedating antianxiety medication, but it takes at least a week to work. The antihistamine-derived agent, hydroxyzine, may also be useful.

Hypnotics

These medications are designed specifically to help the sleepless sleep. Most are highly sedating benzodiazepines, and all can be effective in counteracting insomnia. Yet the hypnotics all are psychologically, if not physiologically, addictive and should be used only for short periods of time, then tapered to avoid withdrawal. They are most useful to cancer patients at the crisis points, such as learning of diagnosis, prior to surgery, or in the immediate aftermath of recurrence.

Alternative or Complementary Medications

These days, any number of pharmaceuticals claiming to have pyschological effects and marketed as safe and natural can be obtained over the counter. Examples are St. John's wort, which is used against depression, kava kava, which is said to be effective against anxiety, and valerian root, which is used to treat insomnia. Some people think that by taking these plant-derived substances they are somehow avoiding the dangers and risks of prescribed drugs. This is a false notion. St. John's wort, kava kava, and valerian root are as much drugs as are Prozac and Valium—that is, all are substances that change the structure and function of living tissue. Some come from the pharmacy, and others from the natural foods store, but they're all still drugs with side effects.

Alternative medications can be helpful. For example, the data suggest that St. John's wort is effective against mild to moderate depression. That much is known. What isn't known is how such herbal remedies interact with many of the medications used in cancer treatment. If you are interested in alternative or complementary therapies, always discuss the issue with your physician *before* taking over-the-counter medications.

Psychotropic Medications Used in Cancer Treatment

Note: Brand names appear first, followed by generic names in parentheses.

ANTIDEPRESSANTS

Tricyclics (TCAs)

Adapin, Sinequan	(doxepin)
Anafranil	(clomipramine)
Aventyl, Pamelor	(nortriptyline)
Elavil, Endep	(amitriptyline)
Norpramin	(desipramine)
Surmontil	(trimipramine)
Tofranil	(imipramine)
Vivactil	(protriptyline)

Selective Serotonin Reuptake Inhibitors (SSRIs)

Celexa	(citalopram)
Luvox	(fluvoxamine)
Paxil	(paroxetine)
Prozac	(fluoxetine)
Zoloft	(sertraline)

Tetracyclics

Asendin	(amoxapine)
Ludiomil	(maprotiline)

Novel, or Heterocyclic, Antidepressants

Desyrel	(trazodone)—good for sleep
Effexor	(venlafaxine)
Remeron	(mirtazapine) —antinausea properties
Serzone	(nefazodone)—good for sleep
Wellbutrin	(bupropion)—energizing

Monoamine Oxidase Inhibitors (MAOIs)

Marplan	(isocarboxazid)
Nardil	(phenelzine)
Parnate	(tranylcypromine)

Stimulants

Adderall	(mixed amphetamines)
Concerta, Metadate, Methylin, and Ritalin	(methylphenidate)
Cylert	(pemoline)
Dexedrine	(dextroamphetamine)
Provigil	(modafinil)—a new stimulant

NEUROLEPTIC MEDICATIONS

Novels (Atypicals)

Clozaril	(clozapine)
Geodon	(ziprasidone)
Risperdal	(risperidone)
Seroquel	(quetiapine)
Zyprexa	(olanzapine)

Typicals

Haldol	(haloperidol)
Loxitane	(loxapine)
Mellaril	(thioridazine)
Moban	(molindone)
Navane	(thiothixene)
Polixin	(fluphenazine)
Serentil	(mesoridazine)
Stelazine	(trifluoperazine)
Thorazine	(chlorpromazine)
Trilafon	(perphenazine)

ANTIANXIETY MEDICATIONS

Benzodiazepines

Ativan	(lorazepam)
Klonopin	(clonazepam)
Librium	(chlordiazepoxide)
Serax	(oxazepam)
Tranxene	(chlorazepate)
Valium	(diazepam)
Xanax	(alprazolam)

Others

Atarax, Vistaril	(hydroxyzine)
Buspar	(buspirone)

HYPNOTICS (SLEEPING MEDICATIONS)

Benzodiazepines

Ambien	(zolpidem)
Dalmane	(flurazepam)
Halcion	(triazolam)
Prosom	(estazolam)
Restoril	(temazepam)
Sonata	(zaleplon)

Others

Benadryl	(diphenhydramine)
Desyrel	(trazodone)
Serzone	(nefazodone)
Somnote	(chloral hydrate)

8

FOR FAMILY AND FRIENDS

LIKE WAVES RIPPLING OUT from a pebble cast into a still pool, cancer affects not only the individual with the disease but everyone and anyone connected to that person. If life has not yet taught you John Donne's compassionate lesson that "no man is an island," cancer surely will. Watching a loved one or close friend battle cancer is a painful experience that powerfully affects the relationship, often forces it in new, sometimes difficult directions, and always offers the opportunity for new depth, intimacy, and connectedness.

Second-Order Patients and Their Reactions

When someone falls ill with cancer, the family is suddenly faced with a whole new set of challenges. They have to provide emotional support, share in gathering information and making decisions about treatment, provide physical care at home, deal with insurance companies, and possibly pay some of the often-staggering medical costs. Even though only the individual with cancer actually has the disease, the psychological effects of the illness extend into the family. Psycho-oncologists often refer to family and intimate friends as *second-order patients,* people who do not suffer from the disease yet are subject to many of the same psychological consequences. For example, people close to the patient usually go through the same sort of numbing, denial, and existential crisis at diagnosis as the patient, suffering the same transient anxiety, sleeplessness, and depression. The emotional cycles of cancer tend to hold as true for second-order patients as they do for the individual with the disease.

For too long, medical professionals treating the disease have tended to consider family and friends as little more than the backdrop against which cancer's drama plays out. Now we are coming to understand that they too are profoundly affected by the disease and as needy of attention and care as the patient.

As we see in Chapter 2, personality style has a great deal to do with how individuals respond to and cope with cancer. The same holds true for family members and friends. People with controlling personalities have a different emotional response than do those with dependent styles. In addition, the reaction to cancer is influenced by one's relationship to the patient, the stage of the disease, and the developmental stage of the family.

Relationship to the Patient

Obviously, one of the most important factors determining the emotional reaction to cancer in a loved one is the relationship to the individual with cancer. Studies of spouses show that they suffer through the same emotional crises as the cancer patients themselves and that their psychological suffering may actually worsen over time. And although spouses share the cancer experience vicariously, often their perceptions of one another are inaccurate. The causes of these emotional misreadings include anxiety, denial, and, paradoxically, love and concern, which under any circumstance affect perception. In the studies, patients typically didn't realize how upset their spouses were over the pain they were suffering, and spouses underestimated the value patients placed on their support. In one study of couples affected by breast cancer, the husbands tended to hide their distress over their wives' suffering, thinking that this strategy provided the best sort of support, but the wives saw their reaction as a sort of insensitive rejection. The effect of this fundamental emotional miscommunication was increased distance in the relationship at a time when greater closeness would have been of more benefit to both partners.

For the parents of cancer patients who are children, the experience of cancer can be utterly devastating. The anguish of having a desperately sick child can strain the healthiest marriages, lead to alcohol and substance abuse, and upset the ability to work and to function socially. Posttraumatic stress symptoms, such as recurrent, intrusive recollections of the child's illness and suffering, nightmares, extreme vigilance, hyperarousal, and detachment, affect a substantial number of mothers and fathers and often last for years beyond the child's illness.

Cancer has profound effects on any child, whether it is a parent or sibling who is sick. Given that the sibling relationship is often full of both identification and rivalry, nurturance and competition, cancer cuts very deep. Some studies show that siblings fare worse than parents. In cases where a parent has the disease, younger children are often left out of the decision-making process surrounding the cancer. Even if they are included, children often worry that they bear responsibility for causing the cancer. They experience grief and yearning for the parenting that cancer is denying them, fear for their own welfare and future, and feel angry and resentful about being abandoned and, in their view, shunted aside. If children do not have a realistic idea of what is going on, they are likely to develop their own explanatory fantasies—which are certain to be more disturbing than the truth itself, however unvarnished. Psychological symptoms, acting out, and school problems can easily develop.

In talking to a child about cancer, consider both your child's chronological and psychological age. The older and more mature a child is, the more he or she is able to handle. Be direct, honest, and realistically optimistic, and follow the child's lead in his or her need to know. Don't tell a child any more than he or she asks to be told. Respect denial if it is working—that is, if the child is not exhibiting symptoms of anxiety or depression. Reassure the child that the cancer isn't his or her fault, that he or she will be taken care of no matter what happens, that all feelings, even the seemingly nasty ones, are acceptable, and that it is appropriate to go on living life and not put everything on hold. There's nothing wrong with continuing to play sports, hanging out with friends, or completing college applications.

The emotional reactions of friends vary with the type and quality of the relationship. In some cases, friendships are more intimate, closer, and longer lasting than family relationships. Then the experience of cancer is devastating and difficult for the friend who feels for the patient with a vicarious emotion much like a spouse's, and experiences a deep, humane sadness that someone so close must endure such a difficult journey. There is fear, too, of death and loss. The friend may even put himself or herself in the patient's role. "If he or she can get cancer, then so can I," says the friend, which rouses in the friend the same sort of mortality crisis that affects the patient. This reaction, in turn, can cause guilt or shame, as the friend assumes himself or herself to be self-centered in the midst of someone else's suffering. What makes the situation even more difficult for friends is that the family tends to draw in around the patient and often excludes friends as outsiders. This isolates the friends and makes it difficult to express their feelings and connect as they need to with the patient.

The good thing about cancer is that it can precipitate growth and maturity in a relationship, enhancing the intimacy or even untangling unhealthy dynamics. That is what happened with Suzanne and her mother, Martha. They never really got along once Suzanne reached adolescence. Ironically, the likely reason was that they were so much alike: strong-willed and stubborn, somewhat aloof and detached. As adults, they were cordial, yet never close.

The situation changed when Martha, then sixty, was diagnosed with chronic leukemia and began chemotherapy. Suzanne, now thirty-eight and a mother herself, felt both shock and sadness at the illness in a woman she considered sturdy and invincible. She wanted very much to be of help. Although resistant at first, Martha, weak and depleted from her treatments, welcomed Suzanne's daily visits. Suzanne often came with her ever-active children and plastic containers full of chicken soup made according to Martha's own recipe.

"It's not as good as mine," Martha said teasingly. "But it'll do."

Martha and Suzanne never spoke openly about their past or even their present, but a cold glass of juice here and a propped-up pillow there exceeded words and spoke of their connection. Cancer had softened a hard relationship between a mother and a daughter, healing and repairing their bond.

Stage of Cancer

The acute phase of cancer—when the disease is first diagnosed and treatment is decided upon and implemented—faces the family with a sudden and overwhelming challenge. Typically, some family members are more distressed than others—a reaction that they may try to hide, only to become increasingly resentful over time at the fact that the other members of the family don't see what a hard time they are having. At the same time, the family usually rallies together, rising to the demands of the moment. However, a conspiracy of silence may develop. Seeking to put the best face on the cancer and its consequences, the family may declare certain topics, concerns, and emotions beyond the pale. This short-term strategy ultimately backfires, because it defeats the need for the truth that intimacy and love demand. Rather, the chance to express feelings—both hopes *and* fears—creates a milieu that allows open communication, which is the basis for meeting the physical and emotional needs of everyone involved.

A contemporary wrinkle during the acute phase is the family's demand that the patient act upbeat and optimistic, even when he or she feels just the opposite. The motivation is good; it comes from the family's concern and love for the patient—even as an unconscious and irrational belief that happiness may cure the cancer—and fear about the outcome of the disease. But the subliminal message the family delivers is, "Look, we're helpless to stop the disease. So it's up to you. And remember: If you get sicker, it's all your fault!" The family demand for optimism paradoxically blames the victim for a disease over which he or she has no control.

In cancer's chronic phase—during the patient's return home after surgery, following long treatments or lengthy hospitalizations, and throughout survivorship, when the disease is in remission—the family's emotional situation changes. During the acute phase, practically all family energy and activity was directed at caring for the patient's needs. In the chronic phase, the needs of the other family members come to the fore again, creating a potential conflict. As time passes, family members often make their anger, jealousy, and needs known. A paradox emerges: Even as the patient is getting better, family members may actually show more psychological symptoms. And since the patient's health has improved, extended family and friends slowly withdraw their support, thinking it is no longer needed. As a result, the family can become socially isolated even though they would welcome assistance. Additionally, the family focus may remain on the cancer, which can put off decisions about other matters, such as getting a child off to college or planning for retirement. In a way, family life can shift into neutral, and little or nothing new happens, except events directly related to the cancer. At the same time, though, the family breathes a collective sigh of relief over the loved one's survival and learns anew to appreciate the small things, such as Sunday dinner or a night at the movies, as gifts and blessings.

Family Developmental Stage

Like individuals who grow from infancy into childhood and adolescence and finally into maturity, families develop through time. In a young family, dealing with cancer may be a greater challenge because family members may lack experience, maturity, or independence. Cancer in one spouse, particularly in a very young marriage with no children, may drive that person back into his or her family of origin, creating tensions between the parents and the healthy spouse. And cancer in a young child is particularly difficult. The parents are trying to care for a child who may die, and they feel guilt, baseless but powerful, over not protecting the child against serious illness.

In a family of middle years, with adolescent or young adult children, the pattern is different. If one of the children is the patient, that person has the age and, potentially, the maturity to understand what can happen, and works to find some kind of meaning in the experience. Although the child is in a life stage where the struggle for independence is the key issue, parents are likely to become overprotective, leading to strain and conflict. If it is a parent who is sick, adolescents and young adults may bow out, avoiding contact with the patient, a behavior that seems callous and indifferent but is in fact a way of dealing with a stress too large for the young person to handle. At times, though, teenagers are capable of remarkable altruism toward the ill.

In an older family, the key issue is the fear one spouse carries about losing the other spouse. The couple feels a strong need for physical contact and closeness, but the lack of privacy in hospitals and convalescent settings makes this difficult to achieve, heightening the stress of the situation. Adult children, accustomed to seeing the parent acting like a parent, find it difficult to deal with the self-absorption and childlike behavior, a function of regression, that is often typical in the sick elderly. Guilt is the usual response. As for grandchildren, they and their grandparents often enjoy a special, warm, and conflict-free relationship. So the fear of loss on both sides can be profound.

How to Support a Cancer Patient

Given that being connected by bonds of family or friendship to an individual with cancer is permeated with such powerful emotions, how is a person to behave? How can one do good rather than harm and ease the situation for all concerned?

In fact, family and friends can do a great deal of good—for themselves and the patient—when both the ill and the healthy keep these psychological guidelines in mind:

- *Care and nurturing is different from creating dependency.* There is a fine but important line between nurturing someone and turning that person into an infantilized dependent. Resist the desire to be controlling or patronizing. Don't overanticipate; follow the patient's cues about what he or she needs. Take over at times when help is needed, such as right after surgery or a chemotherapy infusion, and be prepared to back off as the patient gains strength and his or her neediness decreases. Respect the patient's desire for solitude and privacy. Be sure to involve the patient in all decisions whenever it is possible.

- *Be yourself.* Cancer is a disease, not a demand to reinvent a relationship. As much as possible, be with the patient just as you always have been. To do anything else is only to create a relationship that is as stilted as it is false. It's okay to express negative feelings such as anger, frustration, or impatience. You did so before the patient fell sick; there's no reason to stop now.
- *Banish secrets.* Withholding information backfires. Keeping secrets is stressful, and it cuts other family members and friends off from being able to provide the empathy and closeness the patient needs.
- *Be an advocate.* Go to doctor's appointments and take notes or turn on the tape recorder. Research treatment options. Locate support groups in the area. Provide information in those areas where the patient probably lacks the physical and emotional energy to investigate.
- *Include the children.* You can't keep it from kids anyway. They know something is wrong, and not telling them the truth leaves them wide open to self-manufactured fantasies about their own responsibility for matters that are much worse than reality. Exactly what to tell them, and in what detail, depends on their age and psychological maturity. Be aware of the warning signs that the stress of the situation is affecting children severely enough to require professional help:

  Sleep disturbances, such as waking up during the night, sleepwalking, nightmares

  Eating disturbances, such as eating constantly or very little or overeating at mealtimes

  Abnormal fears, such as of mail carriers, babysitters, and delivery people, being in the same room as the sick person

  Regression, for example, previously toilet-trained child who suddenly wets the bed

  Acting out, such as performing poorly in school, or picking fights with other children

  Physical and psychological withdrawal

- *Listening counts.* You don't have to have the answer, only a willing ear. Just listen when the patient says how he or she feels. If tears come— yours or the patient's—let them flow. Accept whatever the loved one says without judgment or criticism. Your one task is to pay attention.
- *Small things matter.* Surprise the patient with flowers or a CD that you know he or she will love. And a hug always helps.
- *When friends or family ask what they can do to help, tell them.* People want to help, but they don't know what to do. Taking care of tasks such as doing the laundry, walking the dog, or picking the kids up after the game can be a godsend for someone who is acutely ill or undergoing treatment. Ask friends to drive the patient to the radiology laboratory once a week or to cook dinner once a month. Meeting such everyday needs can take a huge burden off the patient and gives others a way to be usefully involved.

The Special Needs of Caregivers

In some cases, especially when cancer is chronic, one family member ends up bearing the major weight of caring for the patient, both psychologically and physically. In adults, this is most likely the spouse or life partner. When a child has cancer, a parent typically fills this role. Sadly, caregivers are often treated like part of the medical equipment in the patient's room, when in fact they are in a terribly stressful and difficult position. Many find their careers stalled or sidetracked, their savings spent, their friends lost. In their way, caregivers need care as much as do the patients to whom they are giving care.

The Caregiver's Bill of Rights, developed originally by the Alzheimer's Association for the caregivers of people with Alzheimer's disease, applies equally well to people caring for cancer patients. If you are a caregiver, consider the following and reread it as often as you need to:

I have the right to make mistakes and be imperfect.

I have the right to forgive myself and begin anew.

I have the right to say no and not feel guilty or selfish.

I have the right to relax.

I have the right to let go of yesterday and embrace today.

I have the right to enlist the cooperation of my family.

I have the right to laugh and be happy.

I have the right to arrange my own priorities.

I have the right to take time for myself.

I have the right to have my needs considered important by others.

I have the right to be free to do special things for myself.

I have the right to take time off even if it costs money.

I have the right to take charge.

I have the right to make decisions when other family members refuse to participate.

I have the right to be self-preserving so that I can take care of others.

Support groups are one of the most important sources of support for those who are caring for people with cancer. Formal and informal support groups for cancer caregivers are excellent props and aids, as Seth, a married, forty-five-year-old, self-employed antique dealer in a New York suburb found out.

Seth had a life that was, if anything, too full. Besides working a never-ending week to keep his business prosperous, he coached his daughters' soccer teams, volunteered at an inner-city homeless shelter, and was an avid Knicks fan. Seth was always overworked but energized by his various involvements.

That all changed when Seth's wife, Danielle, was diagnosed with uterine cancer. Although determined to be the quietly competent hunter who could do anything, Seth soon found himself overwhelmed. It was all he could do to get the kids out of bed and through the door to school, keep his business functioning, and accompany Danielle on each of her many medical appointments. And, as Danielle went through the predictable cycle of emotions accompanying her disease, Seth sat up many nights listening to Danielle's fears and worries and discussing treatment options.

Soon Seth found himself short-fused at work, thin-skinned with his daughters, and uninterested in the Knicks.

One morning while he was sitting in the waiting room of the radiation oncology center where Danielle was receiving her initial treatment, Seth struck up a conversation with another man the same age. It turned out they were both Knicks fans, and both had wives with uterine cancer. The talk soon went from batting averages to their mutual frustrations over being working husbands whose wives had cancer.

"You know," said Seth's newfound acquaintance, "a bunch of us get together for dinner at this little downtown restaurant on Tuesday nights. It's great. The food's good, but the important thing is we can talk about what's going on, and I find it really helps to know I'm not alone in this mess. Why don't you come?"

Seth did. He found it helped him enormously to discover other men in precisely the same situation. He was able to express many of the feelings he had been hesitant to share with Danielle, determine that he was stronger than he realized, and get some practical advice on matters that made his life easier—for example, drafting a couple of other parents to help out as assistant coaches on the soccer team and asking Danielle's mother to fix dinner on Tuesdays so that he could have dinner with the group.

Seth had been trying to do it all, which was bound to result in failure. When he drew a line around what he could do, he gave himself psychological breathing room. Then he made another wise move: He shared the responsibility with others, namely other soccer parents and Danielle's mother. And going out with his group on Tuesdays gave him a much-needed opportunity to unwind and enjoy himself. Seth found that not only did his mood improve, but he was also better able to attend to Danielle when she was in pain or feeling down. In the end, a caregiver who cannot give care to himself or herself can't give care to anyone else either. An important guideline for caretakers is to establish limits of responsibility.

For more information on finding caregivers' support groups, see the Resources section at the end of this book.

When the Death of a Loved One
Is Inevitable

There is no way around it: In the end, we all die. Our culture attempts to deny death, to treat it as abnormal and unexpected. This wrongheaded point of view causes more pain than solace, for it turns us away from the reality that life ends, and prepares us poorly for what will finally happen.

We can take two important psychological actions in the face of death's inevitability. One, the core message of this book, is to live well—to accept each day as a gift, not a right, and to welcome it with gratitude. The other is to accept death when it does happen and be aware of the emotions it precipitates.

The Stages of Grief

In most cases, death from cancer isn't sudden. Rather, family and friends know that the patient is dying. In fact, research studies show that the opportunity to prepare for death makes the grieving process easier for the survivors over the long term than does a sudden, unexpected loss.

Still, when some relatives and friends are told that death is inevitable, they deny this reality, become angry with the medical staff informing them of the true state of affairs, demand that doctors find a cure for the incurable, and refuse to accept what is happening. This can adversely affect the patient, who may then feel an obligation to save his or her survivors from emotions they are unwilling to bear.

Steve, one of my terminally ill patients, was only thirty-six, the father of two, and the vice-president of marketing in a successful company. He had been diagnosed with an unusual and extremely aggressive pancreatic cancer. His life expectancy was measured in months, and there was nothing for his physicians to do except make him comfortable. The characteristic that most struck me about Steve in our initial conversation was his optimism. Successful throughout his life, he saw every hurdle as a challenge he was sure to clear. And that had been true, time and time again, until he contracted cancer. Steve knew full well that he would die soon. He was disturbed less about the inevitability of his death than about his inability to find an optimistic take on what he was going through. As a result, Steve was feeling extraordinarily anxious, the reason his physician asked me to see him on the oncology unit.

"I can't say I'm anxious and worried to my wife or my friends," he confessed. "They expect me to be upbeat. They couldn't stand it to see me down, defeated."

"I wouldn't be so sure," I suggested. "When you really feel your feelings and let others know about them, you are inviting them in. It creates a bond between you. Your attempt to be unfailingly optimistic is isolating you, and that, I suspect, has a lot to do with the anxiety you are experiencing."

Steve said he'd think about it. And he must have, because when I saw him a couple of days later, his wife and two men who turned out to be Steve's closest buddies from high school were laughing and crying together. The atmosphere in the room was charged with both grief and honesty. When Steve died just several weeks later, that honesty on both sides of the bed made closure around his death all the more possible.

Once survivors accept the inevitability of the patient's death, they may begin anticipatory grief—that is, a passage through the phases of grief even before the patient has died. The survivors begin to prepare themselves for the loss and attempt to heal any conflicts still outstanding in the relationship.

Yet, no matter how well-prepared-for and anticipated, the actual death still comes as a potent shock. It initiates the stage of acute grief, which often begins with numbness and denial and is soon followed by waves of distress. Survivors feel agitated, cry easily and sometimes uncontrollably, feel aimless and unfocused, experience a lump in the throat and digestive upset, have significant trouble sleeping, feel weak, sigh, and are preoccupied with images of the deceased. They usually withdraw from their social activities, feel anxious, look very sad, dream or even hallucinate about the dead person, drop into a depressed mood, eat very little or too much, feel distant from friends, and suffer a depleting loss of energy and endurance. Some survivors develop a short-lived abnormal fear of cancer, probably as a way of identifying with the lost loved one. Surviving spouses may feel angry or envious when they see other couples together.

Acute grief is commonly said to last several months. In fact, the length of time varies with the nature of the relationship and the personality of the bereaved person. Despite what you may read, there is no magic number.

At some point, acute grief gives way to chronic grief, which has symptoms very much like a minor to moderate depression. Sleep disturbance, occasional crying, and a low-grade sad mood are the most striking hallmarks. Usually, the greater the distress in the acute stage, the greater the pain in the chronic. And chronic grief also has no definite time limit. One year is a commonly quoted number, but in the case of close and long-lived relationships, symptoms of grief have been found in scientific studies from two to four years after the death.

When Grief Is Problematic and a Cause for Concern

Distinguishing normal grief from abnormal grief is difficult because the symptoms of the latter are largely the same as the former, only more pronounced, prolonged, or extreme. The usual rule with grief is to let it happen. But when certain patterns arise, professional help is wise.

One is the *dependent grief syndrome,* also called *unresolved grief.* In this pattern, the symptoms of acute grief continue indefinitely and fail to give way to the usual signs of chronic grief. The cause is the loss of a loved one on whom the bereaved was extraordinarily dependent. Because the self-esteem, self-confidence, and identity of the survivor was determined by the relationship with the dead person, the survivor is left with a major, untreatable wound from the death. The survivor sees himself or herself as weak, abandoned, and unneeded, with no chance of rescue. Extended mourning gives the survivor a social role and still allows him or her to create a self-definition founded on the dead. It is an unconscious way to boost self-esteem and preserve some of the status he or she is afraid to lose.

More common than dependent grief syndrome is major depression rooted in bereavement, which affects about one out of five survivors. Besides suffering from grief, these individuals are strongly impaired in their ability to function in social or occupational settings, morbidly preoccupied with feelings of their own worthlessness, or so depressed that it is all they can do to get out of bed in the morning. Bereavement is most likely to turn into major depression when the individual has a poor social support system, a psychiatric history of the disorder, and extreme acute grief with depressive symptoms; was highly dependent on the person who died; and is facing other major stressors, such as the loss of a job or other deaths. As might be expected, the death of a child is particularly likely to result in major depression. Depression rooted in bereavement, even around the death of a child, is highly treatable.

It had been two years since the death of her daughter when Randi, then fifty-four, came to see me complaining of depression. Karen, one of Randi's four children, had died when she was twenty, the victim of a sarcoma, an aggressive soft-tissue cancer. Karen had been diagnosed as a high school senior and went through a series of grueling treatments, including a failed bone marrow transplant, over the remaining three years of her life. That ordeal left Randi terribly bereaved, and she dropped into the depths of despair soon after Karen's death. When she came to see me, she had already been through several brief courses of psychotherapy and medication. She remained profoundly depressed despite treatment. Except for suicidal thoughts, Randi suffered from every symptom of major depression.

I soon discovered that Randi had other tragedy in her past. When she was an adolescent, her mother and father died simultaneously in a car accident, leaving Randi to raise two younger siblings as a surrogate parent. She postponed college and a social life until her brother and sister were educated and on their own. Then she married, had four children, and accumulated college credits toward a degree and teaching certification.

In the course of our psychotherapy sessions, Randi came to see how her history as a young woman compounded the grief she was feeling over the death of her daughter. "Let me tell you, though," she insisted, "the death of my parents is nothing compared to the loss of my daughter. There is no way to explain the death of a child."

In fact, I could only begin to imagine the suffering she had been through, and I am sure that my own worst imagination was but a fraction of what she felt. Still, as we worked together, Randi came to understand that she was clinging to her grief as a way of holding on to her daughter. If she gave up her mourning and started to enjoy herself again, she feared she would lose her daughter again. This perception caused her constant anxiety and guilt.

She realized too that her depression was a way of punishing herself. "I can't stop thinking that I should have done more for Karen. There must have been a way to save her. If I'd looked harder, maybe I could have found it."

There was no easy solution to Randi's dilemma, and it took us years to finally untangle her feelings. In the end, she was no longer clinically depressed, although she realized that she would always live with an undertow of sadness. But Randi finally discovered something survivors need: She discovered a place within her for the grief, and, with those emotions safely enshrined in that part of her psyche, she was able to reconnect with family and friends and get on with her now-bittersweet life.

How the Grief of Children Differs

For decades, psychiatrists following the lead of Sigmund Freud believed that children do not experience grief. Freud, we have discovered, was wrong. Children do feel grief, but the emotions vary with the child's age, and they are expressed in ways distinctly different from adult feelings of loss.

Preschool children (three- to five-year-olds) have the most difficulty understanding that death is inevitable, that the lost loved one will remain lost. Once that idea sinks in, they show signs of stress: bedwetting, nightmares, whining, stomachaches, and powerful anxiety when separated from a parent. Children from six to eight years old grasp the irreversibility of death and are likely to see themselves as responsible. They like to tell stories about the deceased and may express a desire to die too—not a suicidal wish, but a childlike expression of grief and a desire to be united again with the lost parent or sibling. Between nine and fourteen years of age, children find their emotions about death overwhelming and attempt to escape them, preferring involvement with school activities or friends over talking about their feelings. Particularly between ages twelve and fourteen, adolescents hate to express grief and act in ways that seem egocentric to adults. By the time they reach fifteen, adolescents act much more like adults in the ways they express their feelings about death, entering an acute phase of grief after the death and moving into chronic grief over time.

What children of any age need most when a parent or sibling dies is open communication with their surviving parents and other important adults. Holding information back, even for their supposed good, compounds the difficulty and makes it that much harder for children to cope.

Making Grief Manageable

Any way you look at it, experiencing the death of a loved one is painful and wrenching, an ordeal to which there is no solution except endurance. Yet, if you pay attention and let the process work its way through, you will survive—changed for sure, but also feeling deeper and more true to yourself.

Here are some guidelines for getting through the experience:

- *Get support from a support group.* Grief eases when it is shared. Support groups help by making grief and loss normal and by reassuring participants that life goes on, albeit changed. A study of widows in support groups found that they did better over the two-year period following the spouse's death than did widows who received no such help.

  Numerous support groups exist to help people in grief, whether parents, spouses, siblings, or friends. Examples are Compassionate

Friends and Candlelighters, which help parents who have lost children. Both groups are listed in the Resources section at the back of the book. Hospitals, mental health associations, and local chapters of the American Cancer Society either run groups or can make referrals.

Support groups don't work for everybody, however. Men especially seem to have difficulty with the kind of emotional sharing upon which group dynamics build. If this is the case, involvement in a church or synagogue is a good alternative.

- *Support yourself.* For some people, recording feelings in a journal, writing poetry, painting, sculpturing, or playing music is helpful. Others find comfort in reading poetry or prose with a spiritual bent, such as the Psalms, the book of Job, the Buddhist sutras, or the writings of William Blake.
- *Let mourning be.* Don't fight it. Feel as bad as you want to, for as long as you need to. Grief has no timeline; don't hold yourself to an artificial schedule. If you're not over it, you shouldn't be.
- *The calendar triggers tough times.* Birthdays, wedding anniversaries, holidays, and the like can bring old feelings of grief back. Let them be bittersweet times, dark and sad with loss and bright with warm memories.
- *Accept change.* Recognize that your life has changed forever. Particularly when a child has died, sadness will always be with you. Don't fight it or judge it. The positive here is that this change may heighten your own awareness of life, opening you to greater meaning and depth than you have felt before.
- *Seek professional help if you need it.* If your distress becomes markedly worse, talk with a mental health professional. A great deal can be done to alleviate emotional symptoms that make grief worse than it needs to be.

9

CANCER'S JOURNEY AND OTHER GOOD FORTUNES

CANCER HAS THE POWER not simply to threaten life but to transform it. This is the paradox of the disease: Even as it puts life at risk, it offers the opportunity to turn that life toward greater meaning. Cancer's journey permits us to focus on what is good and valid, and to reshape what is not. That is the deepest meaning of healing.

What continues to dazzle me in my work with people who go through the cancer experience is that most of them learn both to cope with the illness and to use it as an opportunity to stretch and grow. My patients have taught me that life is not something to be postponed indefinitely. Today's experiences, relationships, longings, and loves cannot be put off until the fantasy of endless tomorrows. Too often, we find ourselves placing life on hold, saying such things as "I'll do that when I have time" or "That's something I'm saving for retirement." Quite apart from the practical needs of making a living, these statements can be nothing more than excuses for ignoring the important things that lie right before us, such as a quiet moment with a spouse or lover, a game of catch with an eager young son, or a gymnastics meet with a daughter.

Paul Tsongas, a Massachusetts senator and Democratic presidential hopeful who lived for years with cancer, once said words that went something like this: "I've never heard of anyone on their deathbed saying, 'I wish I'd spent more time at the office.'" He was stating well how cancer puts a new sense of priority and importance on day-to-day life. When tomorrow is at risk, today counts all the more.

The other fallacy that cancer deflates is the notion that we own our lives—that life is a possession like artwork or jewelry. Rather, cancer has the capacity to drive us toward the wisdom captured in William Blake's lines:

> He who binds himself to a joy
> Does the wingéd life destroy.
> But he who kisses the joy as it flies
> Lives in eternity's sun rise.

We spend much of our lives building structures that we hope will ensure us joy. We earn college and professional degrees, develop careers, buy homes and cars, attempt to amass money and wealth. In trying to make ourselves secure, we often lose a sense of what is important. Cancer provides the force that upends illusion and brings us to the true depth of everyday existence. Yes, our moments are mixed with both joy and sorrow, but we can know each of them in their fullness, even as they take to wing.

As I look back over this book, I am struck again by the way so many of the people I have encountered in my career have made cancer into a turning point:

- Nancy, the nurse and mother with bladder cancer, not only stepped out of her depression, but also came to see that basing her self-esteem solely on what she did for others left her incomplete. Developing a more balanced sense of caring and being cared for, Nancy became happier and more mature.
- At first, Jack saw lung cancer as a just punishment for his longtime cigarette habit. A rigidly moralistic upbringing and a sense that self-worth comes only from external achievements predisposed Jack to guilt. As he gave up that rigidity, Jack came to respect himself more for who he was rather than who he should be. When his cancer went into remission, he felt as if he had begun a new life—which, in fact, he had.

- Roberta, the personal injury attorney whose small breast lump turned out to be cancer, coped well with the expected reactions to her diagnosis by neither demeaning nor criticizing how she felt. She didn't judge her feelings; she just felt them. Often letting feelings be felt, even when they are unpleasant, can prevent emotional disorders.

- Ally reacted to her double mastectomy as is to be expected: She felt mutilated and asexual, unable and unwilling to sustain any kind of erotic connection with her husband, Michael. In therapy, the two of them learned that there is more to sex than a perfect body and that love has many forms of physical and emotional expression.

- Dana's panic disorder served to remind her of the unavoidable reality that we all die. She returned to her life with both pleasure and sadness, understanding that each happy moment is a temporary present, not an endless possession.

- Mary Ann, the flight attendant who developed posttraumatic stress disorder after undergoing a double mastectomy, came to understand that her value consisted of elements besides physical beauty. And her experience demonstrates how psychotherapy and medication can help a person with cancer get through a serious psychological disorder.

- Seth tried to do it all and found he couldn't after his wife, Danielle, was diagnosed with uterine cancer. In fact, the most competent of us can't do it all—and need not. Seth learned that compassion is a state of feeling, not a balance sheet of good deeds done.

The Lessons Cancer Teaches

Over the years that I have been practicing psycho-oncology, I've often reflected on the many insights provided by the remarkable people who cope with this disease. In the end, their wisdom comes down to a better way of living, whether with cancer or without.

- **Life is a brief, bountiful lease, but we don't own it, and we can't renew it indefinitely.** Possession doesn't work. Letting life move through us does. And life follows its schedule, not ours.

- **Everyone can't love us, and everyone won't hate us.** Live your life as you need to, without excessive concern for approval or rejection.

- **Never take a warm embrace or a firm handshake for granted.** Every act of intimacy, no matter how small, brings comfort.

- **What's important changes.** Yesterday it mattered whether the lawn was as green and as well tended as the neighbor's. Today it's irrelevant. And that's just fine.

- **Physical and emotional pain are part of life.** They can be dealt with. Suffering is different; no one needs to bear up under agony. Medication, relaxation techniques, and other treatments can turn the unbearable into the bearable.

- **An active fighting spirit makes each day meaningful.** But different people fight differently. Let yourself challenge cancer in the way you find best.

- **We must let go of irritable indignations and angry competitions.**

- **When awakened by the alarm clock, be grateful, not grumpy.** The morning affirms life.

- **Be generous in how you see yourself.** Most of us try our best even though we don't give ourselves credit for it.

- **Patience, like all else in life, is relative.** Does it really matter if we have to sit in traffic or stand in line at the supermarket?

- **It is remarkably difficult to be fully honest with yourself or others, but the attempt speaks to courage.** Remember that there is no true intimacy without honesty.

- **Find joy in listening.** There's no better way to hear the world.

- **Generations validate goodness.** Grandparents and grandchildren are golden connections of time.

- **Slow down.** Think, feel, smell, taste, and touch. Stay in the moment.

- **Make peace or let go.** Create peace inside yourself and in your relationships. Rid yourself of relationships that drain and deplete, if they can't be fixed.

- **We can all change and evolve.** Every person has the capacity to modify what is wrong with his or her life.

- **Whatever you feel, let yourself feel it.** It doesn't matter whether the emotion is "good" or "bad." The important thing is to experience fully what you are feeling.
- **There is no such thing as too much laughter or too much fun.** Our lives and the world need more of both.
- **Hopefully, work and profession provide meaning.** But the tenacity we bring to such tasks need not negate our chance to play.
- **Respect yourself in what you eat, but don't forget the pleasure of food.** Broccoli and grains are fine, but don't be afraid to let yourself have a bowl of Ben & Jerry's now and again.
- **Our memories should sustain us, not demean us.**
- **Spirituality, regardless of religion, should be pursued.** All religions tap into the same deep well. The goal is to find that still place beneath.
- **Ethics and morality should be an ideal, not a concept driven by guilt.**
- **Seasons turn too quickly.** We need to pay more attention to falling leaves and setting suns.
- **We can all find personal dignity.**
- **Uncertainty and loss of control lie at the center of our living and dying.** The sooner we learn that there are no guarantees, the sooner we can live fully.
- **Friendships and family hold and heal our hearts.**
- **Intimacy and love are the most potent antidotes to darkness.**

A Closing Word

As I have said throughout this book, cancer delivers a potent wake-up call to review and rewrite our lives. No other journey offers a more powerful catalyst for psychological, spiritual, and interpersonal evolution. Cancer encourages us to discover emotional survival in both sickness and health. And, by paying closer attention to this short-term lease called life, our time becomes deep and full.

Ultimately, this is cancer's good fortune.

SOURCES AND FURTHER READING

Benson, Herbert. *The Relaxation Response.* New York: Outlet Book Inc., 1993. A classic book explaining the response as a form of meditation.

Bruning, Nancy. *Coping with Chemotherapy.* New York: Ballantine, 1985. Although an older reference, it still provides a good overview of chemotherapy.

Canfield, Jack, et al. *Chicken Soup for the Surviving Soul: 101 Healing Stories of Courage and Inspiration.* Deerfield, FL: Health Communications, Inc., 1996.

Cotter, Arlene. *From This Moment On: A Guide for Those Recently Diagnosed with Cancer.* New York: Random House, 1999. A collection of brief "wisdoms."

Cousins, Norman. *Anatomy of an Illness.* New York: Dutton, 1989. Cousins, a fine writer and longtime editor of the *Saturday Review,* reveals how he used laughter and humor to survive an illness that his physicians thought was incurable.

Harpham, Wendy. *After Cancer: A Guide to Your New Life.* New York: HarperCollins/Norton, 1994/1995. This comprehensive Q&A-format volume includes a section on the emotional aspects of cancer that focuses on survivors.

Harpham, Wendy. *Diagnosis Cancer: Your Guide Through the First Months.* New York: Norton, 1998. By a physician with a primary focus on medical issues.

Hersh, Stephen. *Beyond Miracles: Living with Cancer.* New York: Contemporary Books, 1998. This book emphasizes taking control of one's course of treatment and touches on the emotional aspects of the disease, acting more as a guide to choosing among traditional and complementary therapies.

Holland, Jimmie, and L. Sheldon. *The Human Side of Cancer: Living with Hope, Coping with Uncertainty.* New York: HarperCollins, 2000. A fine, insightful overview of the emotional aspects of cancer.

Kabat-Zinn, J. *Full Catastrophe Living: Using the Wisdom of Your Body and Mind to Face Stress, Pain, and Illness.* New York: Delacorte Press, 1990. This excellent book, by a pioneer and leader in the field, focuses on Eastern meditation techniques and shows how the practice of mindfulness—living wholly in the moment—can help in coping with disease.

Koocher, G. P., and J. L. O'Malley. *The Damocles Syndrome: Psychosocial Consequences of Surviving Childhood Cancer.* New York: McGraw-Hill, 1981. This book looks in depth at the peculiar and continuing stress that arises from fear that cancer will recur.

Lang, Susan, and Richard Patt. *You Don't Have to Suffer: A Complete Guide to Relieving Cancer Pain for Patients and Their Families.* New York: Oxford University Press, 1994.

Lazarus, R., and S. Folkman. *Stress, Appraisal, and Coping.* New York: Springer, 1984. A classic work describing the principles and types of coping.

LeShan, Lawrence. *Cancer as a Turning Point.* New York: Plume, 1989. Focusing on the mind-body connection, LeShan offers a method for physicians to incorporate into their practices.

Love, Susan. *Dr. Susan Love's Breast Book.* Cambridge, MA: Persus, 2000. A comprehensive overview of breast care and disease.

Moyers, Bill. *Healing and the Mind.* New York: Doubleday, 1993. An adept and respected journalist interviews experts on mind-body medicine and investigates how their ideas and techniques can work against disease and toward enhanced quality of life.

Nessim, Susan, and Judith Ellis. *Can Survive: Reclaiming Your Life After Cancer.* Boston: Houghton Mifflin, 2000. General advice about survivorship.

Siegel, Bernie. *Love, Medicine, and Miracles: Lessons Learned About Self-Healing from a Surgeon's Experience with Exceptional Patients.* New York: Harper/Perennial Library, 1990. A surgeon's best-selling book describing his program for instilling hope in cancer patients.

Spiegel, David. *Living Beyond Limits: New Hope and Help for Facing Life-Threatening Illness.* New York: Times Books, 1993. Drawn from Dr. Spiegel's excellent research on the benefit of support groups for terminally ill breast cancer patients, this book charts an approach to living fully while facing up to a chronic, fatal illness.

MEMOIRS

Albom, Mitch. *Tuesdays with Morrie.* New York: Bantam, 1997. A relationship forms between professor and writer as the former teaches the latter about living life fully and dying with dignity.

Armstrong, Lance, with Sally Jenkins. *It's Not About the Bike: My Journey Back to Life.* New York: Putnam, 2000. A memoir by the world-class athlete who came back from metastatic testicular cancer to win the Tour de France, bicycle racing's most difficult competition, two years in a row.

Grealy, Lucy. *Autobiography of a Face.* New York: Harper Perennial, 1994. A poet's memoir of dealing with a disfiguring cancer of the jaw as a child, adolescent, and young woman.

O'Connor, Mary Bradish. *Say Yes Quickly: A Cancer Tapestry.* Comptche, CA: Pot Shard Press, 1997. A collection of poems, mostly sonnets, and short prose pieces about living with cancer.

Rosenbaum, Edward. *A Taste of My Own Medicine.* New York: Random House, 1988. A doctor diagnosed with cancer describes his difficult shift into the world of patients. This book was the basis of the film *The Doctor*, starring William Hurt.

Sontag, Susan. *Illness as Metaphor.* New York: Farrar, Straus, & Giroux, 1978. A highly acclaimed cultural and literary critic, herself a cancer survivor, Sontag dissects the metaphor of cancer as the product of emotional repression.

DEATH, DYING, AND GRIEF

Attig, Thomas. *How We Grieve: Relearning the World.* New York: Oxford University Press, 1996. The author is the former president of the Association for Death Education and Counseling.

Bourard, Marguerite. *The Path Through Grief: A Compassionate Guide.* New York: Prometheus, 1998.

Kübler-Ross, Elizabeth. *On Death and Dying.* New York: Macmillan, 1969.

Rich, Phil. *The Healing Journey Through Grief: Your Journal for Reflection and Recovery.* New York: Wiley, 1999. Informational guide for using writing as a means for healing.

Schiff, Harriet. *The Bereaved Parent.* New York: Penguin, 1977. Classic book on the loss of a child.

Van Praagh, James. *Healing Grief: Reclaiming Life After Any Loss.* New York: Dutton, 2000. A spiritual view of grieving.

MEDICAL TEXTBOOKS ON CANCER

Abeloff, M., et al., eds. *Clinical Oncology.* 2nd ed. New York: Churchill Livingston, 2000.

DeVita, V., et al., eds. *Principles and Practices of Oncology.* 5th ed. Philadelphia: Lippincott-Raven, 1997.

Holland, J., et al., eds. *Cancer Medicine.* 4th ed. Baltimore: Williams and Wilkins, 1997.

Murphy, G., et al., eds. *The American Cancer Society Textbook of Clinical Oncology.* Atlanta: American Cancer Society, 1995.

MEDICAL TEXTBOOKS ON PSYCHO-ONCOLOGY

Holland, Jimmie, ed. *Psycho-oncology.* New York: Oxford University Press, 1998. The standard text for mental health professionals on psycho-oncology.

Rundell, J., et al., eds. *The American Psychiatric Association Textbook of Consultation-Liaison Psychiatry.* Washington: APA Press, 1996. A general text that looks at psychiatric aspects of medical illness.

Strain, J., and S. Grossman. *Psychological Care of the Medically Ill: A Primer in Liaison Psychiatry.* New York: Appleton-Century-Crofts, 1975. The seminal work on understanding the psychological impact of medical illness.

SCIENTIFIC STUDIES AND ANALYSES

Chochinov, Harvey Max, Keith G. Wilson, Murray Ens, et al. "Desire for Death in the Terminally Ill." *American Journal of Psychiatry* 152 (1995): 1185–1191.

Fawzy, Fawzy I., Nancy W. Fawzy, Christine S. Hyun, et al. "Malignant Melanoma: Effects of an Early Structured Psychiatric Intervention, Coping, and Affective State on Recurrence and Survival 6 Years Later." *Archives of General Psychiatry* 50 (1993): 681–689.

Friedman, Howard S., and Gary R. VandenBos. "Disease-Prone and Self-Healing Personalities." *Hospital and Community Psychiatry* 43 (1992): 1177–1179.

Geringer, Edith S., and Theodore A. Stern. "Coping with Medical Illness: The Impact of Personality Types." *Psychosomatics* 27 (1986): 251–261. A useful analysis of how different personality types react to serious disease.

Gray, Ross E., Margaret Fitch, Catherine Phillips, Manon Labrecque, and Karen Fergus. "To Tell or Not to Tell: Patterns of Disclosure Among Men with Prostate Cancer." *Psycho-oncology* 9 (2000): 273–282. A study of men treated for prostate cancer with prostatectomy shows that they avoided disclosure of their illness whenever possible for a variety of reasons, including a low perceived need for support, fear of stigmatization, the need to minimize the threat of cancer as a way of coping, the desire to avoid burdening others, and the realities of the workplace.

Greer, Steven, T. Morris, and K. W. Pettingale. "Psychological Response to Breast Cancer: Effect on Outcome." *Lancet* 2 (1979): 785–787.

Holland, Jimmie C., and Sheldon Lewis. "Emotions and Cancer: What Do We Really Know?" In *Mind-Body Medicine: How to Use Your Mind for Better Health*, edited by D. Goleman and J. Gurin. Yonkers, NY: Consumer Reports Books, 1993.

Levinson, James L., and Claudia Bemis. "The Role of Psychological Factors in Cancer Onset and Progression." *Psychosomatics* 32 (1991): 124–132.

McCaul, Kevin D., Ann K. Sandgren, Brenda King, et al. "Coping and Adjustment to Breast Cancer." *Psycho-oncology* 8 (1999): 230–236. Study showing that women who used an avoidant coping style suffered more distress than women who employed other strategies.

Spiegel, David. "Can Psychotherapy Prolong Cancer Survival?" *Psychosomatics* 31 (1990): 361–366. An excellent summary and overview of the possible connection between therapy and increased survival time.

Spiegel, David. "Efficacy and Cost-Effectiveness of Group Psychotherapy for Patients with Cancer." *TEN* 2 (2000): 56–61. This paper makes the case that group therapy helps cancer patients adapt better and increases quality of life.

Spiegel, David, J. Bloom, H. C. Kraemer, et al. "Effect of Psychosocial Treatment on Survival of Patients with Metastatic Breast Cancer." *Lancet* 2 (1989): 888-891. The paper in which Dr. Spiegel and his research group first reported that survival might be prolonged by group therapy.

Spiegel, David, and Catherine Classen. *Group Therapy for Cancer Patients: A Research-Based Handlbook of Psychosocial Care.* New York: Basic Books, 2000.

Stein, Sara, Kaye Hermanson, and David Spiegel. "New Directions in Psycho-oncology." *Current Opinion in Psychiatry* 6 (1993): 838–846.

Weisman, D. "Early Diagnosis of Vulnerability in Cancer Patients." *American Journal of Medical Science* 271 (1976): 187–196.

Wellisch, David K., Alisa Hoffman, Sherry Goldman, et al. "Depression and Anxiety Symptoms in Women at High Risk for Breast Cancer: Pilot Study of a Group Intervention." *American Journal of Psychiatry* 10 (1999): 1644–1645. A study finding that group therapy helps reduce emotional distress in women at increased risk for breast cancer.

RESOURCES

AMERICAN ACADEMY OF PAIN MEDICATION
  4700 West Lake Avenue
  Glenview, IL 60025
  847-375-4777
  www.painmed.org

Dedicated to understanding and managing pain and providing referrals to physicians with expertise in pain control.

AMERICAN BRAIN TUMOR ASSOCIATION
  2720 River Road, Suite 146
  Des Plaines, IL 60018
  800-886-2282
  www.abta.org

Information, treatment explanations, support resources, and research updates for brain tumor patients and their families.

AMERICAN CANCER SOCIETY
  1599 Clifton Road, NE
  Atlanta, GA 30329
  800-ACS-2345
  www.cancer.org

A nationwide community-based voluntary health organization dedicated to eliminating cancer as a major health problem by preventing the disease, saving lives, and diminishing suffering from cancer through research, education, advocacy, and service. A variety of service and rehabilitation programs are available to patients and their families. The Web site offers tools to help patients evaluate treatment options.

AMERICAN FOUNDATION FOR UROLOGIC DISEASE/PROSTATE CANCER SUPPORT NETWORK

www.afud.org

The foundation's Prostate Cancer Support Network links prostate cancer support groups, survivors, families, and friends by developing grassroots advocacy, bringing increased national awareness to the issues of prostate cancer, and coordinating awareness and advocacy programs, with a special emphasis on the issues of prostate cancer survivors.

AMERICAN INSTITUTE FOR CANCER RESEARCH

1759 R Street, NW
Washington, DC 20069
202-328-7744
www.aicr.org

The nation's third largest cancer charity and a pioneer in the area of diet and nutrition as they relate to the prevention and treatment of cancer. AICR has helped encourage innovative research on diet, nutrition, and the prevention and treatment of cancer, while also serving as one of the country's leading sources for educational programs for cancer prevention.

AMERICAN LUNG ASSOCIATION

1740 Broadway
New York, NY 10019
212-315-8700
www.lungusa.org

Dedicated to preventing lung disease, including lung cancer, and promoting lung health through programs such as anti-tobacco campaigns.

AMERICAN PAIN SOCIETY
    4700 West Lake Avenue
    Glenview, IL 60025-1485
    847-375-4715
    www.ampainsoc.org

Dedicated to understanding and managing pain and providing referrals to physicians with expertise in pain control.

AMERICAN PSYCHIATRIC ASSOCIATION
    1400 K Street, NW
    Washington, DC 20005
    888-357-7924 or 202-682-6000
    www.psych.org

Provides referrals to psychiatrists who have expertise and interest in working with cancer patients experiencing emotional difficulties.

AMERICAN PSYCHIATRIC NURSES' ASSOCIATION
    1200 19th Street, NW, Suite 300
    Washington, DC 20036
    202-857-1133
    www.apna.org

Provides referrals to nurses who have expertise and interest in working with cancer patients experiencing emotional difficulties.

AMERICAN PSYCHOLOGICAL ASSOCIATION
    750 First Street, NE
    Washington, DC 20002
    202-336-6080
    www.apa.org

Provides referrals to psychologists who have expertise and interest in working with cancer patients experiencing emotional difficulties.

AMERICAN SOCIETY OF PSYCHOSOCIAL AND BEHAVIORAL ONCOLOGY/AIDS

www.ipos-aspboa.org

Promotes the psychological, social, and physical well-being of patients with cancer, AIDS, and allied diseases and of their families at all stages of disease and survivorship through clinical care, education, research, and advocacy.

BURGER KING CANCER CARING CENTER

4117 Liberty Avenue
Pittsburgh, PA 15224
412-622-1212
www.trfn.clpgh.org/cancercaring

Helps cancer survivors, their families, and concerned friends cope effectively with the emotional impact of cancer through a variety of free support services, including professional counseling; support groups; a telephone help line; Live Well with Cancer programs and workshops; the Jewish Healthcare Foundation Resource Library, featuring hundreds of books, brochures, and audio- and videotapes; age-specific support for children who have a family member with cancer; age-specific bereavement groups; Look Good Feel Better, an award-winning self-esteem program for female survivors; and community support groups in the Pittsburgh metropolitan area.

CANCER CARE, INC.

1180 Avenue of the Americas
New York, NY 10036
212-221-3300
www.cancercare.org

Dedicated to providing emotional support, information, and practical help to people with cancer and their loved ones through a toll-free counseling line, teleconference programs, office-based services, and the Internet. All services are free of charge and available to people of all ages, with all types of cancer, at any stage of the disease, and to their family members and caregivers.

CANCER RECOVERY FOUNDATION

P.O. Box 238

Hershey, PA 17033

800-238-6479

www.cancerrecovery.org

A resource for information on conventional, complementary, and alternative cancer treatments and a provider of psychological and spiritual counseling, with a focus on treating the whole person: body, mind, and spirit.

CANCER RESEARCH INSTITUTE

681 Fifth Avenue

New York, NY 10022

800-992-2623 or 212-688-7515

www.cancerresearch.org

Dedicated to fostering the science of cancer immunology, which is based on the premise that the body's immune system can be mobilized against cancer. The institute has supported nearly a thousand scientists and clinicians at leading universities and research centers worldwide.

CANCERVIVE

1875 Century Park East, Suite 600

Los Angeles, CA 90067

310-203-9232

www.cancervive.org

Dedicated to improving the quality of life for cancer survivors. The group provides emotional support, education, and advocacy to assist survivors through one-on-one and telephone counseling nationally.

CANDLELIGHTERS CHILDHOOD CANCER FOUNDATION
7910 Woodmont Avenue, Suite 460
Bethesda, MD 20814
800-366-2223
www.candle.org

Provides emotional, educational, and practical support to children with cancer and their families, and promotes awareness of childhood cancer and the need for childhood cancer education and research.

CAREGIVER SURVIVAL RESOURCES
www.caregiver911.com

Books, workshops, and other aids to help caregivers cope with the demands of caregiving.

CHEMOTHERAPY FOUNDATION
183 Madison Avenue, Suite 403
New York, NY 10016
212-213-9292

Stimulates and accelerates innovative therapies for the control, cure, and prevention of cancer through basic research, clinical studies, and improved application techniques; improves the education and expertise of practicing oncologists through symposia and publications; educates patients and the public in the progress and promise of chemotherapy. The foundation sponsors selected research projects at seven major metropolitan medical centers and conducts an annual international symposium for professionals.

CHILDREN'S ONCOLOGY CAMPS OF AMERICA
75 Richland Memorial Park, Suite 203
Columbia, SC 29203
803-434-3533

CITY OF HOPE NATIONAL MEDICAL CENTER

1500 East Duarte Road
Duarte, CA 91010
626-359-8111
www.cityofhope.org

A National Cancer Institute–designated comprehensive cancer care center that focuses on research, education, outreach, and information. City of Hope is a founding member of the National Comprehensive Cancer Network, which develops and institutes standards of care for cancer treatment.

COMPASSIONATE FRIENDS

P.O. Box 3696
Oak Brook, IL 60522-3696
630-990-0010

Helps resolve grief following the death of a child and provides information to help others be supportive.

COPING MAGAZINE

P.O. Box 682268
Franklin, TN 37068-2268
615-790-2400
e-mail: copingmag@aol.com

A periodical devoted to helping readers cope with the physical and emotional aspects of cancer.

CORPORATE ANGEL NETWORK

Westchester County Airport, Building 1
White Plains, NY 10604
914-328-1313
www.corpangelnetwork.com

Provides free air transportation for patients flying to and from recognized cancer care centers in the United States by arranging for patients to use empty seats on corporate aircraft making business flights.

CURE FOR LYMPHOMA FOUNDATION

215 Lexington Avenue
New York, NY 10016-6023
800-CFL-6848 or 212-213-9595
www.cfl.org

A nationwide not-for-profit organization dedicated to funding research and providing support and education for patients with Hodgkin's disease and non-Hodgkin's lymphoma and their families.

ECAP

Exceptional Cancer Patients
2 Church Street, South
New Haven, CT 06519
www.ecap-online.org/home.htm

The official Web site for Bernie Siegel, M.D.; also provides a useful listing of Internet links.

I CAN COPE

c/o American Cancer Society
1599 Clifton Road, NE
Atlanta, GA 30329
800-ACS-2345

Provides emotional support and education for patients and their loved ones primarily through group meetings.

INTERNATIONAL MYELOMA FOUNDATION

125650 Riverside Drive, Suite 206
North Hollywood, CA 91607
800-452-CURE
www.myeloma.org

A nonprofit organization dedicated to improving the quality of life for multiple myeloma patients while working toward prevention and cure. The foundation aims to help patients, families, friends, caregivers, and the medical community.

LEUKEMIA AND LYMPHOMA SOCIETY

1311 Mamaroneck Avenue
White Plains, NY 10605
800-955-4572
www.leukemia-lymphoma.org

Dedicated to fighting blood-related malignancies, such as lymphoma, leukemia, and myeloma. The group supports research, provides services to patients, and increases public awareness of these diseases.

LIVING BEYOND BREAST CANCER

10 East Athens Avenue, Suite 204
Ardmore, PA 19003
610-645-4567
Survivors Helpline: 888-753-LBBC
www.lbbc.org

A nonprofit educational organization committed to empowering all women affected by breast cancer to live as long as possible with the best quality of life. Programs include semi-annual educational conferences, a quarterly educational newsletter, outreach to medically underserved women, a consumer-focused educational booklet, the Paula A. Seidman Library and Resource Center, Young Survivors group, the Survivors Helpline, and a Web site.

NATIONAL ALLIANCE OF BREAST CANCER ORGANIZATIONS

9 East 37th Street, 10th Floor
New York, NY 10016
212-889-0606
www.nabco.org

An information and education resource on breast cancer as well as a network of more than four hundred member organizations nationwide. NABCO provides information to medical professionals and their organizations and to patients and their families, advocates for beneficial regulatory change and legislation, and helps connect women with needed services.

NATIONAL ASSOCIATION OF SOCIAL WORKERS

750 First Street, NE, Suite 700
Washington, DC 20002-4241
202-336-8200
www.socialworkers.org

Provides referrals to social workers who have expertise and interest in working with cancer patients experiencing emotional difficulties.

NATIONAL BONE MARROW TRANSPLANT LINK

20411 West 12 Mile Road, Suite 108
Southfield, MI 48076
800-LINK-BMT
comnet.org/nbmtlink/index.html

This educational organization for BMT patients provides information about the treatment process, including the logistics of bone marrow transplantation, finances, and medical insurance; it also offers a peer support program.

NATIONAL BRAIN TUMOR FOUNDATION

785 Market Street, Suite 16
San Francisco, CA 94103
800-934-CURE
www.braintumor.org

Provides information and support for brain tumor patients, family members, and health care professionals and supports innovative research into better treatment options and a cure for brain tumors. The Web site provides objective information regarding treatment options, community resources, and opportunities for patients, caregivers, family members, and health care providers to support each other.

NATIONAL BREAST CANCER COALITION
  1707 L Street, NW, Suite 1060
  Washington, DC 20036
  202-296-6854
  www.stopbreastcancer.org

A national grassroots organization that seeks to eradicate breast cancer through advocacy and action.

NATIONAL CANCER INSTITUTE CENTER
  Information Service
  Building 31, Room 10A16
  9000 Rockville Pike
  Bethesda, MD 20892
  800-4-CANCER
  www.cancernet.nci.nih.gov

Conducts and supports research, training, health information dissemination, and other programs with respect to the cause, diagnosis, prevention, and treatment of cancer, rehabilitation from cancer, and the continuing care of cancer patients and their families. NCI is part of the federally funded National Institutes of Health

NATIONAL CANCER SURVIVORS DAY FOUNDATION
  P.O. Box 682285
  Franklin, TN 37068-2285
  615-794-3006
  www.ncsdf.org

Supports hundreds of local hospitals, support groups, and other cancer-related organizations that hold National Cancer Survivors Day events by providing guidance, education, and networking. NCSD is an annual nationwide celebration of life held in more than seven hundred communities to honor the 8.4 million Americans who are surviving cancer.

NATIONAL HOSPICE ORGANIZATION

1901 North Moore Street, Suite 901
Arlington, VA 22209
800-839-3288
www.nho.org

An organization dedicated to ensuring the physical and emotional comfort of seriously and terminally ill patients. Services, including effective pain management by nurses with advanced training, are often provided in patients' homes as well as in skilled health care facilities. There are numerous local chapters throughout the country.

NATIONAL LYMPHEDEMA NETWORK

1611 Telegraph Avenue, Suite 1111
Oakland, CA 94612
800-541-3259 or 510-208-3200
www.lymphnet.org

Provides education and guidance to lymphedema patients, health care professionals, and the general public by disseminating information on the prevention and management of primary and secondary lymphedema, a common complication among cancer survivors. The NLN seeks to standardize quality treatment for lymphedema patients nationwide and supports research into the causes and possible alternative treatments. NLN provides a toll-free information line, referrals to treatment centers, a newsletter, educational programs for health care professionals, a biennial national conference, and an extensive computer database.

NATIONAL MARROW DONOR PROGRAM

3433 Broadway Street, NE, Suite 400
Minneapolis, MN 55413
800-MARROW-2
www.marrow.org

Facilitates unrelated-donor stem cell transplants for patients who do not have matching donors in their families, no matter what their racial or socioeconomic background.

NEW JERSEY CANCERCARE

241 Millburn Avenue, Suite 241-C
Millburn, NJ 07041
800-813-4673
and
141 Dayton Street, Suite 204
Ridgewood, NJ 07450
201-444-6630

Regional affiliates of Cancer Care, Inc. that provide resources similar to those of the national organization.

PATIENT ADVOCATES FOR ADVANCED CANCER TREATMENTS

1143 Parmelee, NW
P.O. Box 141695
Grand Rapids, MI 49504
616-453-1477
www.prostatepointers.org/paact/

An educational support organization for men with prostate cancer and their families.

THE SKIN CANCER FOUNDATION

245 Fifth Avenue, Suite 2402
New York, NY 10016
800-SKIN-490
www.skincancer.org

Conducts education campaigns, encourages early detection, supports research into new diagnostic techniques and therapies, and focuses attention on melanoma, the most life-threatening skin cancer.

SUPPORT FOR PEOPLE WITH ORAL AND HEAD AND NECK
CANCER, INC.

PO Box 53
Locust Valley, NY 11560
516-759-5333
www.spohnc.org

An educational and support organization for people with head and neck
cancer. The group provides a telephone support line, a newsletter, and a
survivor-to-survivor support network.

THE WELLNESS COMMUNITY

2716 Ocean Park Boulevard, Suite 1040
Santa Monica, CA 90405
310-314-2555
www.la.wellnesscommunity.org

Helps cancer patients fight for recovery along with their physicians and
other health care professionals in the hope that their efforts will have a
positive effect on the course of the illness.

Y-ME

National Organization for Breast Cancer
212 West Van Buren, 4th Floor
Chicago, IL 60607
800-221-2141 (800-986-9505 for Spanish speakers)
www.y-me.org

Trained counselors who have had breast cancer provide information and
support. Access to a variety of resources is offered twenty-four hours a day.
Trained male counselors are also available to talk to male partners of
breast cancer patients. Up-to-date information is provided on approved
mammogram facilities, comprehensive breast centers, treatment and
research hospitals, and support programs nationwide.

INDEX

ABOUT THE AUTHOR

Roger Granet, MD, FAPA, has practiced psychiatry for twenty-five years, focusing much of his work on the emotional issues faced by cancer patients. Dr. Granet serves as a consulting psychiatrist at Memorial Sloan-Kettering Cancer Center, clinical professor of Psychiatry at Weill Medical College of Cornell University, lecturer in psychiatry at Columbia University College of Physicians and Surgeons, attending psychiatrist at New York Presbyterian Hospital-Cornell division, and director of consultation-liaison psychiatry at Morristown Memorial Hospital. The author of numerous medical journal articles and textbook chapters, Dr. Granet has also published essays in the *New York Times* and two collections of poetry. He is the co-author of four popular books on emotional disorders: *If You Think You Have Depression* (Dell, 1998), *If You Think You Have Panic Disorder* (Dell, 1998), *Is It Alzheimer's? What To Do When Loved Ones Can't Remember What They Should* (Avon, 1998), and *Why Am I Up, Why Am I Down: Understanding Bipolar Disorder* (Dell, 1999). Dr. Granet maintains private practices in Morristown, New Jersey and in New York City.